K.C. Hitchcock
3149 Queens Chapel Rd
#103
Mt Reinier, Md. 20822

NATUROPATHIC PRACTICE

NATUROPATHIC PRACTICE

A valuable guide to students and others in the Principles and Practice of Nature Cure

by

JAMES HEWLETT-PARSONS

(Fellow and Secretary of the Register of Consultant Herbalists and Homoeopathic Practitioners and former Vice President of the Guild of Naturopaths and Osteopaths)

ARCO PUBLISHING COMPANY, INC.
New York

Published 1969 by ARCO PUBLISHING COMPANY, INC.
219 Park Avenue South, New York, N.Y. 10003

Library of Congress Catalog Number 69-14962

Arco Book Number 668-01879-8

PRINTED IN GREAT BRITAIN

CONTENTS

Page

Preface 13

Introduction 15

PART I—THE PHILOSOPHY OF HEALTH AND LIVING

1. First Principles and Axioms 19
   Health 20
   Disease 22

2. The Basic Causative Factors of Disease 24
   Acute disease 24
   Chronic disease 25
   Factors in healing 26
   Methodology 26
   Constructive forces 27
   Life 28

3. Medicaments 31
   Varying concepts of disease 32
   Human development and periodicity 34
   Vital force and eternal youth 35
   Premature age and senility 37
   Education 38

4. Physician Heal Thyself 40
   Division of the cause of disease 40
   Secondary causes of disease 42
   Immunity to disease 43
   Cure 43

5

Healing crisis 44
The principles for which we stand 45

5. Man—the Microcosm: Man—the Macrocosm 47
   Air—Water—Earth—Fire 47
   Rhythm 48
   Light 48
   Earth 49
   The cardinal elements 49
   Omnilateral application 50
   Philosophy and practice 50
   Observation and method 51
   Diagnosis 51
   Prognosis 51
   Pathology 51
   Treatment 52

PART 2—DIETETICS

6. Food Reform 53
   The function of food 54
   Food classification 55
   Proteins—fats—carbohydrates 55
   Proteins 56
   Nitrogen loss 57
   Amino acids 57
   Fats and carbohydrates 58
   Fats and obesity 58
   Cane sugar 58
   Cellulose 59
   Hydrolysis and condensation 59
   Fats and oils 59
   Fats and vitamins 60
   The balanced diet 61

7. Minerals 62
   Mr. Five per cent 62

The principal elements 62
Potassium 62
Sodium 63
Calcium 63
Phosphorus 63
Magnesium 63
Iron 64
Sulphur 64
Silicon 64
Chlorine 65
Therapeutic uses 65

8. The Trace Elements 67
Copper 67
Manganese 68
Cobalt 68
Chromium 68
Silica (to preserve youth) 68
Herbal sources 71
Food supplement 71
Food sources 71
The vitamins 72
Two vitamin categories 73
The oil soluble vitamins 73
Vitamin "A" 73
Vitamin "D" 74
Vitamin "E" 75
Vitamin "K" 75

9. The Water Soluble Vitamins 77
Vitamin "B_1" and "B_2" complex 77
Riboflavine (lactoflavine) 77
Nicotinic acid 78
Pyrodoxin 78
Pantothenic acid 79
Biotin 79
Inositol and choline 79

Para-amino benzoic acid 79
Vitamin "C" 80
Vitamin "P" 82

10. The Ductless Glands 83
     The pituitary gland 84
     The pancreas 84
     The gonads 84
     The ovaries 84
     Adrenal medulla 85
     Cortex 85
     Thyroid 85
     Parathyroid 85
     The thymus, pineal body and spleen 85

11. Treatment by Fasting 86
     The fast 86
     Alterative effect 87
     The initial effects 87
     The enema 87
     Baths and body frictions 88
     Duration of the fast 88
     Restricted diet 88
     General uses of the fast 89
     Practitioners' instructions 90
     Food temperatures 90
     Specialized diets and treatments 90
     The Schroth cure—history 91

12. The Schroth Cure 95
     The importance of diet 95
     Foods to avoid 96
     Drinks 96
     The diet chart (general) 97
     A Schroth dry day 99
     The strict treatment 100
     The true wet pack treatment 100
     Schroth strict regimen 101

13. Mono Diets 103
    The grape cure 105
    The orange diet 106
    Vegetable mono diets 106
    The acids of fresh fruits 107
    More fruits and vegetables and their uses 107
    The milk diet 110
    Yogurt, sour milk and buttermilk 112

14. The All-Meat Diet 114
    Modifications 116
    Fish 116
    Naturopathy and vegetarianism 116
    Unfired foods 118
    Quantitative diet 119

PART 3—HYDROTHERAPY

15. Water: Internal and External 122
    Conditions of treatment 122
    Father Kneipp 123
    Water temperatures 124
    Period and effect 125
    Types of treatment 125
    Internal water treatments 126
    The Epsom salts bath 126
    Sauna or steam baths 127
    Hot baths 128
    Warm baths 129
    Cool baths 129
    Cold baths 129
    Soap and baths 129

16. The Water Jet 131
    The Sitz bath 131
    The whole body pack 131
    The local wet pack 132

Colonic irrigation 133
The value of herbs 135
Epsom salts irrigation 136
Sea salt 136
Iodine 136
Sulphur baths 137
Pine baths 137
Castor oil enema 137
Stomach lavage 137

PART 4—PATHOLOGY AND DIAGNOSIS

17. Pathology 139
Individual cells 140
Leucocyte cells 140
Functions 141
Cell reproduction 141
Pathological cell division 141
Cell uses 142
Classification of disease 143
Survey of pathological conditions 144

18. Naturopathy and Symptomology 147
Etiology 147
Co-ordination 149
Mental state 149
Excesses 150
Pots and pans 150

19. Diagnosis 151
Physical examination 151
Carrying out physical diagnosis 152
The lungs 154
General physical examination 154
Indications of signs observed 155
The vertebrae 156
Organs and parts—spinal nerve centre 156
Taking the body temperature 157

Chemical analysis 158
Prognosis 159

PART 5—PHYSIOTHERAPY

20. Massage 160
    The movements of massage 162
        Effleurage 162
        Frictions 163
        Petrissage 163
        Tapotement 163
        Vibrations 164
    Contra indications 165

21. Medical Electricity 167
    Electricity 167
    Insulators 168
    Treatments 169
        Galvanism 169
    Static electricity 170
    High frequency 170
    Diathermy 171
    Sinusoidal 171
    Ultra violet rays 172
    Radiant heat 172
    Infra red 173
    Ultra sonic 173
    Chromotherapy 173

22. Conclusion 175
    Final notes and advice 175

    Glossary 181

    Index 185

The rays of heaven, the pulse of earth,
Have brought the humble herb to birth;
Its deepening roots in mould will cling,
To bring its blossom to the Spring.
A little rain, a little sun,
So is the wond'rous task begun,
By God designed for man to be
From pain, disease, and hunger free.
In every leaf a healing balm,
In every flow'r a happy charm,
A natural blend of stars and dust,
Pervading all implicit trust.
And if we living could but trust like this,
On mortal life would shine immortal bliss.

J. H.-P.

PREFACE

For many years the Nature Cure profession has felt the need for an up-to-date, all embracing, guide to its practice. Those books which have been, and still are available are for the most part out of date in respect of modern findings in relation to human nutrition.

This book has been designed to meet the needs of students, practitioners and the intelligent layman in all the main branches of Natural Therapeutics which are usually embraced under the general heading of Naturopathy. It includes sections on Dietetics, Hydrotherapy, Fasting, Vitaminotherapy and the specialty treatments such as The Schroth Cure, Mono Diets and various Eliminative Diets. It contains valuable information discovered in recent years concerning the role of the various micro-nutrients such as trace elements, filtrate factors, Vitamins and food synergists which play so important a part in individual health.

It is based on the teachings of the recognized "Masters" of Naturopathy such as Dr. Henry Lindlahr and is thus devoid of many of the present day unilateral ideas usually associated with "Nature Cure" which in recent years has become so pronounced as to give its adherents the epithets of "food faddists" and "cranks". It is broadly based on all those early teachings which followed so faithfully the careful observations of the first practical medical men who became famous from the fifth century B.C. in classical Greece and whose leader, Hippocrates, still enjoys a unique fame, justly earned, throughout the world and whose name remains, after the passage of over two millenniums, a household word.

The proper study of this book will, I feel, widen the horizon of every reader and pave the way for wider and more detailed study of any particular branch of Nature Cure which may catch and hold the reader's imagination. The original tenets of Naturopathy offer a philosophy of living and a system of medicine which, I believe, can be of inestimable benefit to every human being. Prevention of disease, with which Nature Cure is so much concerned, is far better than the spending of large sums of money in attempts to cure—which is rather like closing the stable door after the horse (one's health) has bolted. I do not attempt to "put the clock back" to the crude days of illiterate living "next to nature"—I have tried to show how the individual can live in harmony with his surroundings and remain well, enjoying a long, healthy and vigorous life in a modern civilized, intellectual society. After all, man is a very adaptable animal.

I feel that the fact that you have commenced to read this book proves that you are passionately interested in these things and I welcome you as a reader and hope that as a result of your study of the following pages you will be stimulated to lead a fuller life and to be of ever greater help to those who may seek your advice or follow your example.

J. HEWLETT-PARSONS

INTRODUCTION

It is necessary, before the reader commences the serious study of Naturopathy, that the writer explain certain fundamental concepts on which this book is based. Naturopathy has a very large following of committed vegetarians and the Food Reform and Naturopathic Movement in this country has very strong ties with vegetarianism. And while in this book consideration is given to many non-vegetarian diets which the writer considers in some cases to be absolutely necessary for the health of certain individuals, this is not to say that the vegetarian way of life is to be decried. Animals are our friends and they look to humans to be their guardians, especially in these days of the abominable battery systems of egg production and chicken breeding, not to mention the intensive breeding systems carried on with regard to cattle, and the employment of such a wide range of dangerous antibiotics used in the rearing and fattening of animals for consumption as meat by us humans.

Integrity of human tissue is basically dependent on protein and while many vegetarians can and do secure an adequate amount of first class protein by way of dairy produce, mushrooms, etc., some tend to rely too much on the starches for nutrition, resulting in a serious omission of vital protein. This serious defect in some vegetarian diets can be as conducive to ill health as any indiscriminate and irrational meat eater's diet. The chemistry of the living body depends fundamentally on protein from which it is able to manufacture most of the nutrient it needs with very few exceptions.

There is no doubt that in the foreseeable future the ingenuity of man will have solved the problem of producing readily assimilable first class protein from plant sources but until that time comes it may be necessary in some extreme cases to prescribe an "all-meat diet", while in others an "all-fruit diet" may be indicated. In this book I have made use of our present day knowledge on these subjects, but in all cases where the vegetarian principles of patients are involved, it will be the practitioner's duty to advise accordingly and thus avoid the psychological disturbances which could follow any advice which would run counter to a patient's deeply felt principles on the matter of meat eating.

On the question of Fasts there are also extremists and just as moderate or long fasts may sometimes be indicated, so too will they be contra-indicated in those cases which display such nutritional deficiencies that only the correct nutrient intake will be beneficial.

One other point should be clarified, and this is concerned with that magic word "organic". This is used by the food fads to explain that only living vegetation is of any use as food and that, for example, Vitamin "C" (ascorbic acid) found in an orange is preferable to that found in a tablet which has been synthesized in the laboratory. The word "organic" literally means "organized" so that when Vitamin "C" is taken in an orange it is organized with other vitamins and food factors in a definite way. When it is taken in a blackcurrant it is still "organized" in a definite BUT different way with other factors; BUT the Vitamin "C" itself is exactly the same substance and has exactly the same molecular structure as when it occurs in the orange or the blackcurrant. This should help dispel the erroneous belief held by some that Vitamins isolated in the laboratory are not good food factors. Sometimes in cases of extreme deficiency it is highly beneficial to prescribe large doses of certain nutrients in order to restore the patient to health and vitality as soon as possible—and this after all is the primary object of any kind of treatment. This is where the vitamin or mineral tablet can often be of use. Do not from this infer that naturally grown food is to be deplored—this is the ideal for the already fit in order to keep and preserve health. It is merely postulated here that there is a strong case for the use of concentrated food factors in counteracting perhaps years of nutrient deficiencies with manufactured vitamin and micronutrient tablets to redress the balance of this loss as quickly as possible.

PART I

THE PHILOSOPHY OF HEALTH AND LIVING

FIRST PRINCIPLES AND AXIOMS

Naturopathy is a way of life as well as a system of healing. If its principles are absorbed by the individual consciousness and then operated by the subconscious, they will form a basis for healthy, intelligent living in any chosen sphere of human activity. If they are allowed to dominate the consciousness there is the possibility of the individual becoming a crank or a "food fad" or even a hypochondriac. This, of course, can happen with any subject with which the human mind becomes obsessed. Naturopathy as a philosophy is omnilateral in its approach to life and is not more concerned with the bread you eat than the thoughts which occupy your mind. Only the harmonious balance between the physical, mental and psychic attributes of self can produce true health. Although this book is more concerned with the physical aspects of Naturopathy, the mental and psychic aspects must not be forgotten as it is only by the balanced integration of all three aspects of human life that health can be properly restored in a patient.

Naturopathic Practice is based on laws and principles which, by their application, affect life and death; health and disease. It is a system of healing which if correctly applied will restore the sick without resort to suppressive and harmful drugs. The aim is to rebuild the human being in harmony with his surroundings—physical, mental and psychic. Unless a practitioner can do this, no permanent or lasting result will be forthcoming. The balance must be such that the individual will be inviolate as far as the destructive principles are concerned. In fact, if the preconditions of health are provided in all spheres, the way is paved for the complete recovery of the patient. All the self-repairing processes on every plane of human activity will combine to bring about a restoration of health, it being only necessary thereafter to abide by those same laws in order to preserve and maintain health throughout a long and active life.

The underlying philosophy of Naturopathy properly understood and applied with logical and intelligent methodology will succeed when all other methods have failed. Indeed, how often have we heard of the so-called miracle "cures" effected by properly qualified practitioners of this all-embracing system of healing. All-embracing because, in effect, it is a system which includes such therapies as Herbal Medicine, Homoeopathy and Osteopathy. This was very well understood by Dr. Henry Lindlahr who pioneered Nature Cure in the United States. Many of those lesser than he who came after, have condemned such natural healing arts as Herbal Medicine and Homoeopathy but let us not forget that this great pioneer did in fact embrace these different systems of healing in his philosophy and practice of Nature Cure.

Naturopathy, like Homoeopathy, is concerned with the VITAL FORCE. In disease conditions the basic idea is to stimulate the Vital Force until harmonious balance between the many aspects of individual life has been restored. This is achieved by detailed attention to every aspect of living, for example, by regulating breathing, bathing, eating, drinking, working, resting, leisure and social, sexual and mental activity. On the harmonious balance of all these things depends the health of Man.

Health

We may say then that HEALTH is the harmonious vibration of ALL the elements and forces, physical, mental and psychic, which compose the individual entity ACTING IN HARMONY with all the constructive principles of nature which surround and are external to as well as being an internal part of that life. This concept of health allows for varying conditions of vibration which are external to the human entity and to which the human entity must be attuned if he is to survive in this world and at the same time lead a healthy, positive life. Health is not something for which we all must hope but something which we can all expect as of right. In so many cases man is his own worst enemy in this respect. We spend a great deal of time and study on how best to feed our race horses, or under what conditions our motor car will last longest and give us the best service. We often ignore ourselves and expect to carry on under any or all conditions without thought as to what may be best for the human mechanism.

Study is made of anatomy and physiology, of pathology and disease conditions, but very seldom is any attempt made to co-ordinate the many aspects of our knowledge of man into one broad picture. We live in an age of specialization—something the brilliant Greeks of a bygone age would certainly have opposed. We are a microcosm in a macrocosm and true and lasting health can only be obtained by a complete knowledge of the whole of life—of ourselves in our surroundings. We must never forget this, particularly when dealing with patients, when our powers of observation and our ability to investigate the many facets of the patient's life will be of the utmost importance. The conditions of perfect health in one part of the world may be quite different from those in another and equally, the regimen required of the individual for the maintenance of health in one place may be very different from that required in another. We must not therefore condemn for instance, the diet of the Eskimo (if we are strictly vegetarian) before we have investigated the full facts and found out the reasons why the Eskimo over many centuries has lived well on an all-meat diet and only lost his health when the white man arrived with processed foods of all kinds to trade for seal skins. The Eskimo has paid a very high price for the white man's patronage in this respect.

Disease

Disease is the abnormal vibration of the many aspects of the human entity which can occur on any of the planes mentioned earlier. From this it will be evident that although all disease may be curable, it may not be possible to cure every patient. It is always possible that some deep-seated abnormality may be present on the psychic plane which will only be restored to harmonious balance over many decades or even after many lives. Here the Theosophists have a strong point when they postulate that man ascends an evolutionary ladder covering many lives while the causes effected in one life may not be worked out until the passage of many lives. Whether or not this is true, it is certain that there will be a percentage of patients who for some reason cannot be cured. This is not to say that help cannot be given, but a complete and lasting cure is not possible due to factors beyond our control as they occur outside the orbit of our present finite existence.

Naturopathy is opposed to the allopathic classification of disease. Allopathic medicine classifies disease according to the symptomology presented by the patient. This classification may serve as a rough guide in assessing a disease condition and in eliciting just how abnormal and out of harmony is the individual vibration. Disease means literally DIS-EASE—out of ease. Naturopathy, far from being concerned with a tabulated symptomology, investigates the underlying cause responsible for the upset in the basic harmony of the individual. It is the basic abnormal vibration which has to be changed and restored to normal before health can be regained. The practice of Naturopathy therefore deals with all those factors which have been found to affect the VITAL FORCE beneficially in order that the self-repair processes of the body may be brought into action and relief and cure effected as early as possible. The symptomology is NEVER repressed but quite often is encouraged for Naturopathy believes that the symptoms are the results of the body's own, often feeble, effort to get rid of the underlying causes. If this is assisted by stimulation of the Vital Force, only good can result. However, before we can feel competent to undertake this work, it is essential that we know something of, and understand, the laws involved. In the pages of this book it is intended to put as clearly and thoroughly as possible the principles in so far as they affect the work of anyone whose task it is to help the sick back to health. A good practitioner is a competent practitioner and a practitioner who is competent is confident in himself and in his ability to help the greatest number of patients who may seek his help. The following chapters will gradually unfold the whole philosophy of Naturopathy and provide the armaments with which to cure disease and with which to educate patients so that for ever after they can enjoy ever increasing health without fears of an old age beset with disability. In other words, a long, active and useful life which is only possible to the healthy.

Apart from providing instruction in the practice of Nature Cure, it is hoped that each chapter will provoke and stimulate the reader's own thought so that he will be persuaded to use his own mind in thinking over for himself the many problems and aspects of life which are presented. No book is worth its salt if it is intended only for parrot-like absorption. A book is only useful for study in so far as it provides the reader with a basis for individual thought and action based upon concepts taken up and further analysed. Individual recognition and close acquaintance with a subject produces within the individual a deeper knowledge and insight of the subject studied.

CHAPTER 2

THE BASIC CAUSATIVE FACTOR OF DISEASE

The primary cause of disease is a violation of natural law, which produces a loss of harmonious vibration in all the facets of individual life, thus bringing about a reawakening of the Vital Force. This is the only true cause of disease recognized by the Naturopathic philosophy, with the exception, of course, of personal accident or injury resulting from surgical interference or the prolonged continuance of the individual in an atmosphere which of itself is conducive to death, either by poisoning or suffocation.

The accidental assimilation of fatal poison would be included in the heading of injury resulting from accident. The wilful assimilation of poison which brings about suicide would be the end process of some chronic mental or psychic disease finally manifesting on the physical plane of life and thus completing the cycle to produce death. The only incurable disease for us is death.

Loss of Vital Force produced by violation of natural law results in a lowered vitality with a consequent abnormal composition of blood, lymph and other body tissues, and the accumulation of waste matter and highly toxic substances in the organism.

We can sub-divide the diseases produced by the primary cause into two broad categories :

1. Acute disease.
2. Chronic disease.

Acute Disease

This is always brought about by the violent efforts of the body's own self-repair processes in a supreme endeavour to free the organism of morbid matter, waste products and all other harmful materials. In reality it is a cleansing effort on the part of the body, and at this stage the Vital Force which produces this violent reaction is always fairly strong, and if treatment is prompt and effective, the Vital Force will be stimulated and encouraged in its work until success is the result. If, on the other hand, acute disease is neglected, rapid deterioration can take place with perhaps fatal consequences, or if the Vital Force can sustain the attack but is not strong enough to complete its work nor yet weak enough to succumb, the case will become chronic.

Chronic Disease

Although as pointed out above, this can be an end process of disease, it is not necessarily so. It may not follow an acute outbreak. It may be the result of years of accumulated toxic waste in the system. It may be the result of congenital deficiencies or a congenital impairment of vitality.

You may ask why a chronic case can occur without there being a primary acute affection. Toxins and morbid matter under certain circumstances may gradually and without sounding the alarm bell of "acute disease" gain a position of predominance in the body which can only result in chronic disease. One of the preconditions necessary for this, as already stated, could be congenital factors which, in every case treated, must not be overlooked. We do not propose to go into the teachings of Hahnemann in respect of the miasms, for this rightly comes under the heading of Homoeopathy and is dealt with elsewhere, but the reader would be well advised to become acquainted with the basic rudiments of this study, which is closely linked with the basic ideas of Naturopathic philosophy.

In modern practice, is is the chronic case which more often presents itself for treatment. There is a tendency to think (on the part of members of the public) that acute disease is better cured with a suppressive drug and this attitude is to be deplored. People must be educated and repeatedly told that the skill of the Naturopath is no less with acute disease than with chronic afflictions. In this way Naturopathy would have a lot less cases which have been given up elsewhere and the patients would benefit by having the correct constructive treatment at once, thus saving themselves a great deal of needless suffering and not least, save themselve the many, often harmful, side effects of modern drug medication.

Factors in Healing

There are two main factors in healing. First there is the DISEASE CRISIS. This in effect is the acute reaction resulting from a preponderance of disease conditions over the forces of health (the forces of law and order—of harmonious vibration).

Secondly, there is the HEALING CRISIS which is the former in reverse. A preponderance of the forces of good gain a victory over the accumulated toxins in the body. This is the road to recovery and as such is to be encouraged in every possible way. In doing this you are making practical application of the underlying philosophy of Naturopathy. There are several ways of doing this :

Methodology

Firstly, let us repeat. In order to achieve a cure, it is our aim to restore the patient to harmonious vibrations within himself as well as to make sure that he is in harmony with the totality of his environment.

We restore normal conditions in every way possible. To do this, we make use of the laws of nature which govern these things, and which, by virtue of their constructive principles, cannot fail if given the best possible conditions in which to work. Our practical methods then will be :

1. To restore normal environment whenever required and this includes natural habits of living.
2. To regulate the patient's breathing and restore this to a proper rhythm.
3. To regulate and organize the patient's diet. To supervise the quantity and quality of the nutrients required for the particular case with which we are dealing.

4. To administer wherever indicated natural medicaments which will assist the Vital Force to do its work with ultimate success and without suppressive and harmful side effects.

5. In the prosecution of all of the above we shall enlist the patient's help in an intelligent way and awaken his own sense of personal responsibility so that he will be able to help himself and will not be left in the dark as to what is happening or as to what he may expect during treatment.

If the above methods are properly and skilfully used, only good can result to the patient and the following natural sequels looked for :

Constructive Forces

These methods will bring about the following constructive proccsscs which may be briefly described :

1. They will conserve the Vital Force.

2. They will eliminate toxins and waste and all morbid matter from the system by promoting elimination without injurious or harmful effects.

3. They will build up and improve the quality of the blood by supplying it with all the essential nutrients necessary to health. The blood being the life stream of the body, will carry these nutrients to every tissue of the body in the same way in which it will remove the toxins and waste. All the bodily tissues will be restored to harmony with each other. We must remember that when one organ or part of the body is out of harmony with the rest, then the WHOLE OF THE BODY IS ILL for EACH PART OF THE BODY IS INTERDEPENDENT ON EVERY OTHER.

The previous statement is in small capitals for a purpose, for it is in this respect perhaps more than in any other that the Naturopathic system of medicine differs from the Allopathic.

If your appendix gives you trouble, allopathic medicine will remove it and tell you that you have been "cured" of appendi-citis. Think a moment—is this really true? What has hap-pened? The trouble maker has been removed. Can it therefore ever function again in complete harmony with the rest of the body? Of course not. Never again can the whole organism function in harmonious health; at best this is a bit of patch-work and is not a constructive way of restoring health. No repair is ever accomplished by taking out a broken part and throwing it away as far as the human body is concerned. We know it is possible to live without an appendix and a good many other things, BUT IT IS NOT POSSIBLE TO EVER LIVE IN THAT PERFECT HARMONIOUS STATE OF VIBRATION WE CALL HEALTH WITH ONE OF OUR PARTS MISSING OR EVEN WITH A PLASTIC REPLACEMENT.

Disease is negative and health is positive. If life is carried on in a negative way, then disease will be the result. It is a negation to defy the natural laws of living—to go without fresh air, without pure water and the correct intake of nutrients—early senescence and death will be the result. It is a negation in place of the foregoing to substitute diesel fumes, tobacco smoke, artificial synthetic foods, alcohol etc. without exercise—these will produce suffering, disease and early death. There is no artificial, chromium-plated way to health through some hospital doorway. Health never came out of a hospital, only disease belongs there. Health comes only as a result of man's co-operation with the natural forces of construction—by his conscious observance of natural law and his living in constant harmony with his surrounding vibrations and his innermost forces. THERE IS NO OTHER WAY.

Life

Having considered the aspects of the human organism in health and disease, and having drawn certain conclusions as to the preconditions of these opposing forces in the living body, it remains for us to consider the third over-riding circumstance of our being. LIFE itself. We do know a great deal about life, and we have observed life in a great many of its manifestations during the whole history of the human race and each successive civilization has contributed its own original thought to this great mystery.

We must however realise that in contemplating LIFE, we are contemplating an infinity and we are doing this from a finite standpoint. From a logical point of view this is not possible. The finite cannot comprehend the infinite. This is true also in a relative sense. For example, a human being is a complete totality in a relative sense—he is a universe to himself—he has within his orbit a vast network of communications. He can, for instance, will his finger to move and he can comprehend its movement from his own "infinity". Conversely though, the finger which moved cannot comprehend the "infinite" force which willed it so. It remains a finite part of the "infinite" whole. So the human being in the wider infinity remains a very finite part and in no way able to comprehend the great infinity from the human standpoint. In talking of LIFE in this context we are not merely referring to physical life which is of course finite and only a part of cosmic or infinite life. It was probably a belief in cosmic or infinite life as an extension of physical life which caused Socrates in his prison cell to make that last sublime experiment and take his cup of hemlock.

The nearest we can get to a comprehension of "infinity" is to use the term "Vital Force". This is that part of each human, and in fact that part of each cell of conscious life, which is on terms as it were with the great infinity. The nearer in accord the individual is to infinity, the greater the state of harmony between him and the COSMOS and therefore the greater the chance of his having and keeping a high degree of health. At the ending of a finite earthly existence no doubt this Vital Force continues to function within its etheric membrane, a part then of the greater consciousness as the drop of water is a part of the ocean.

We have been concerned here with something of the metaphysical aspect of our existence. This concept is far from new— such phrases as "man cannot live by bread alone" or its equivalent are as old as the human race, and if we are to be good practitioners of Naturopathy, we must realize that diet alone is not enough. However important our diet and material surroundings may be, we must never forget that we also live in the midst of unseen mental and psychic forces which are equally important to our health and well-being. The many aspects of existence must be co-ordinated and understood as far as possible if we are to be useful to our patients and render good and useful service to our fellow men.

Older civilizations than ours placed the stress on mental and psychic life. We in our present age place the emphasis on material wealth and all that goes with it. Neither of these are true concepts of living, and it is difficult when living in an age of one extreme to pull away and try and take the impartial standpoint when all aspects of life will assume equal importance, but this is the successful way.

The Greek in the Golden Age of Athens during the fifth century B.C. probably came nearer to the ideal of human life than any race before or since. In that astonishing classical epoch men knew the value of complete all-round living. Here in this first and only true democratic community of men, the beauty of the physical form was revered only because it was indeed the house of and vehicle through which was mani-fested the amazing intellectual genius and a phenomenon of psychical rapport which has never again been achieved. In that brief period of human enlightenment, there lived at the same time some of the world's most outstanding dramatists, architects, sculptors, philosophers and scientists—BUT these men were not specialists. It was said that in this remarkable age the "gods" half revealed themselves to men—this perhaps was another way of saying that in that age as never before or since man had a true knowledge of his mental and psychic life which through the centuries that have followed has become dark and clouded. Also remember that in the immediate period following this age Hippocrates lived and founded the first logical system of medicine based on a close observation of man in nature. This as distinct from the older, more stylized schools of medi-cine such as were current in Egypt before man leapt out of the darkness to grasp LIFE in all its aspects freed from the fetters of fear and superstition.

CHAPTER 3

MEDICAMENTS

There is a school of Naturopathy which teaches that under no circumstances must a remedy of any kind be given. This teaching in no way conforms to the accepted instruction of the great pioneers of the movement, and we believe it to be as extremist as allopathic drug therapy and, from the resulting deficiency which could take place, just as dangerous.

The so-called "straight" naturopath will prescribe, in fact insist on, vegetables in his patient's diet but will under no circumstances prescribe, for example, a herbal remedy. This in our view is a rather silly standpoint to take, particularly in view of the fact that the wild herbs are in many cases a more "natural" product than the forced crops of vegetables which abound today. They are naturally composted in the hedgerows and therefore very rich in organized natural nutrients. We advocate the use of herbal remedies in all cases where these are indicated. Their therapeutic virtues are widely known and in a later chapter some information will be given on various herbs where their use is indicated in specific cases.

Homoeopathic medicines also form a valuable part of the Naturopathic system of medicine and healing, and the founder of Homoeopathy, Samuel Hahnemann, was very highly praised by Lindlahr in his works of Natural Therapeutics. Here we must state at once that for the purpose of this book we use the word "Naturopathy" for that branch of Natural Therapeutics which deals with the general adjustment of the individual regimen to conform to natural laws employing non-suppressive medication. Among those Natural Therapies we may list the following : Osteopathy (treatment by manipulative techniques), Physiotherapy, Herbal Medicine, Biochemistry, Homoeopathy,

Psychotherapy and Hydrotherapy. All these therapies employ natural forces in a constructive and harmless way whereby, whatever happens, only good can come to the individual who follows any one or more of them.

Natural medicines (that is herbal remedies, biochemic and homoeopathic remedies) are completely in accord with the constructive principles in nature. They stimulate the Vital Force. They promote elimination and proper assimilation of vital food factors. They promote neutralization of toxins and morbid matter. They promote a Healing Crisis and do not suppress the symptoms.

Varying Concepts of Disease

In Chapter 2 we outlined the basic causative factor of disease. There are many other concepts of disease, some of which oppose our naturopathic idea and some which are relative parts of the whole statement. Care must be taken not to condemn any concept of disease before serious thought has been given to it, using our basic statement as the yardstick by which to measure.

Allopathic medicine is sadly at variance with our own ideas and yet in some respects not so widely different. It will place the causes of disease under many headings, and some of these headings are in complete conformity with the naturopathic standpoint. In these only the methods of treatment vary. Allopathic medicine maintains that GERMS CAUSE DISEASE and under the classification of germ producing diseases come all the infections and contagious diseases and the plagues which beset mankind. Naturopathy on the other hand claims that GERMS ARE THE RESULT OF DISEASE.

These two opposing ideas spring from the minds of two very famous men in the world of medicine. The one, Louis Pasteur, who, as a result of isolating certain germs or bacteria, stated that these were the cause of certain disease conditions in man. The other, Becheaump, also a Frenchman, claimed that the germs isolated by Pasteur were in reality the "scavengers" which invaded the body in an effort to rid it of the accumulated waste products and other morbid matter which were producing a lowered vitality.

We may decide that neither of these men was completely accurate if we think the matter over for ourselves. Let us consider a moment.

In order for the germs to be able to attack the human body, they must have been able to survive before descending on the waste products they have ostensibly come to remove. In the case of infectious diseases, the germs live in the atmosphere and indeed they seem to live in the purest atmospheres. From this we may deduce that they do not live only on morbid matter and the toxins in a sick human. Given that the bacteria can attack even the healthiest human being, what can be our standpoint? It is this—whilst admitting this fact, we can also be very sure that when the attack is against the healthy type with a strong Vital Force, there will be an *acute attack*. The result of this is a foregone conclusion. The germs are rapidly disposed of and absorbed by the armies of phagocite cells which the body marshalls at once to its defence. The use of the correct remedy to stimulate the Vital Force even further, coupled with an adherence to the correct regimen will produce rapid defeat and in fact the result will be a future immunity to this particular germ, as the body in its wisdom will have manufactured the necessary antibodies to secure itself against further attack for some time to come.

Allopathic medicine also subscribes to the fact that there are deficiency diseases, and in this we are in agreement; only our method of treatment is different. The allopath will prescribe massive doses of crude chemicals to rectify the deficiency. Naturopathy contends that the biochemistry of the body is so subtle that in many cases this will cause further suffering, and the crude chemical in any case will not be properly assimilated into the cell structure of the body. Some chemicals, like iron, when prescribed in crude doses, even have the effect of leeching the body of its available natural iron with more disastrous after effects for the patient. Biochemists now know that iron, for instance, needs a synergist in order to effect correct proportional assimilation.

Naturopathy therefore treats deficiency diseases in a far more constructive way than allopathy, and if we think back, this is in strict accordance with the vibratory forces of the body. The body's rate of vibration is far higher than that of crude mineral substances, and if these are prescribed, the vitality will be lowered in an effort to raise the rate of vibration of the crude drug for assimilative purposes. Prescribe only in homoeopathic or biochemic potency or in natural organic (organized form). Herbal remedies contain natural concentrated micro-nutrients in the perfect balance in which the body requires them. That is why they are so useful. Allopathic medicine will isolate alkaloids from these plants, for example quinine is isolated from the cinchona bark, and when so isolated can produce harmful side effects in the human being. Given in its original context—that is organized with all the other natural substances that form part of the plant cinchona—only beneficial results will ensue.

Human Development and Periodicity

We have said that health is living in harmony with the surroundings and maintaining internal harmony of the individual vibrations. The progress of the individual through the various life cycles is governed also by certain general harmonies of development, and we may, as Lindlahr does, refer to this as the LAW OF SEVENS.

It is generally known that our rhythm of life undergoes a change every seven years, and these seven year periods mark the growth, expansion, settlement, decline and ultimate death of the individual. Our modern society makes use of this in using twenty-one as the age of attaining one's majority. In other words, by then the main growth periods have been accomplished. The period between the ages of 28 and 35 is probably the most unsettled and the most unsettling and it is the safe passage through this period that decides in large measure the harmony and stability of the periods which are left. This, and the very first seven years of life.

If the individual survives this period and emerges with the advantages of a previous history of harmonious living in accord with himself and his surroundings, he can look forward to many periods of expanding intellectual and psychic growth with a more or less stable physical body which permits and even assists in his advance into the higher spheres of living.

Vital Force and Eternal Youth

Eternal youth and the concept of everlasting life on earth have dominated man since very early times. It was in particular the preoccupation of the mediaeval alchemist and was the means of founding many of the secret orders. It is even said that there are those few individuals who have wrested these secrets from nature and who have learned to understand her laws so well that they are able to carry on their individual physical lives just so long as they wish. This may indeed be possible, but for the majority of mankind, death is inevitable and this too is the result of an immutable law of nature.

It is also said by some scientists that there is no real reason why a man should die, but always the main reason for the cause of death is given as the body's inability to dispose of morbid matter and waste products. These, it is said, clog the system and in time bring it to a standstill. In other words, if we could secure a state of perfect assimilation and perfect elimination in perpetuity, we should live on earth for ever. The power of the cells to multiply and reproduce themselves *ad infinitum* would go on for ever.

This theory, however, needs a great deal of thought, especially in the light of our previously stated LAW OF SEVENS. We believe it is this law which governs our ultimate death and makes continual life on earth, at any rate for the great mass of humanity, a total impossibility.

This is where our complete harmony comes in. Some say also that the Vital Force is responsible for keeping us young as well as healthy. This is NOT so. The Vital Force is expendable itself and again in complete harmony with the Law of Sevens. If we live intelligently and in harmony with natural law, our Vital

Force will do its work and maintain us in full health and vigour for all our days. It will not preserve us physically for eternity. Our vigour will decline with the succeeding cycles when the periods of stable maturity are over. It is true that the cell structure possesses the power of sub-division and reproduction, and this is why the body can repair itself, but with each renewal, and this renewal goes on whether or not replacement is necessary, there is a subtle difference. This is the real difference between youth and age. We can be perfectly fit whether we are young or old BUT WE CANNOT REMAIN YOUNG under our present pre-conditions of life.

Actually it is from our growth period that we can determine to what kind of age we may expect to live and experiments were carried out in America in recent years during which the growth rate of rats was retarded. This was done by cutting down supplies of nutrition so that just enough was available for the continuance of life but nothing was available for growth. It was estimated from these experiments that if growth were delayed one year during infancy a seven year added expectancy of life may be anticipated in the adult.

One of the reasons why we cannot hope to achieve eternal youth is the fact that body proteins show a gradual change over the years and from having the capacity to remain young and plump, retaining moisture, they dry up and wither producing in extremities that look which can only be described as being between that of a nutmeg and a withered apple. Probably the circulatory system is the most prone to the ageing process and it is a fact that our vitality and length of life are conditioned by some of the smallest factors of the circulatory system—the capillaries. Every nutrient which the cells of the body require, all the oxygen etc., and in addition all the waste products MUST be either taken up or given out by the capillaries. We are back to perfect elimination and perfect assimilation— the balance of perfect health.

Many examples, taken from other forms of life on earth, are cited in proof of the theory that the growth rate determines the length of the life span and some scientists and researchers go so far an to say that when all growth has ceased, then life will end. It is mainly in the sea kingdom among the cold blooded creatures that we have the examples of long life with continued growth. The turtle's age can be judged by its size. Among the mammals on land is the tortoise, which can live to anything from 120 to 200 years. But this subject is, of course, too vast and deep to go into at any length. It is a study in its own right. It has merely been my intention here to stimulate the reader's thoughts on these matters so that he can use his own powers of reasoning and perhaps take up this age-old quest himself. After all, we do have a personal stake in trying to remain alive with good health and vitality for the longest possible time.

Premature Age and Senility

From the previous paragraph it must not be supposed that age of all kinds is natural and inevitable. There is no doubt that under the stresses and strains of modern civilized (so-called) life, with all its faulty habits of living in general, man does age more quickly than he should. Look around you and see how many of your friends of thirty and over are going bald, have greying hair, are fat and podgy, have poor skin, dull eyes, and are forever complaining of many and varied aches and pains, having been to the doctors over periods of years for one complaint or another and into hospital for the removal of this or that. In fact, many will recount their hospital adventures with glee and enthusiasm—they think they are quite unique specimens. THEY ARE NOT. The unique specimen today is the truly healthy and all-round balanced individual. The many live in a rut. They are content to be NOT COMPLETE. They live in pigeon holes with unilateral interests and able to do only one job of work.

The very few are the healthy all-rounders who live well, can do most things reasonably well, can work with their hands with reasonable skill and can work with their minds with comparative skill. These few were the many in the Golden Age of Greece. Socrates was the greatest philosopher who ever lived—the most sublime of men—and yet apart from having so great a mind, he did not neglect his body and could work and enjoy sport with the next man. He could go and fight with his hands in the wars when his beloved city, Athens, was threatened and he could discourse with the greatest minds of any age in the Athenian Agora.

Education

This is the great difference between modern times and the glorious days of life in ancient Greece. In those days men lived longer, with health and vigour of mind and body, into the true sunset of earthly life. Aeschyllus wrote his greatest drama when he was over eighty years of age, and he was one of a whole galaxy of famous names who lived at that time and who lived a full, all-round life with undiminished health to the end. It will repay us to study the reasons for this and compare this state of affairs with our own times.

It will pay us also while doing this to remember that man achieved in those times such high standards in art, culture, politics, building, medicine, philosophy, science, literature and in general living that have seldom if ever been surpassed. Heraclitus in those wonderful years B.C. even postulated an atomic theory. Where did these great minds obtain their education? Certainly there was no "Oxbridge" for them. No great public schools and other centres with a standardized system of teaching which enforced learning along unilateral lines. We are told today that our children suffer from overcrowded classes, from lack of teachers and obsolete buildings. Were these things rectified, we are told, our children would be able to go forward extending the frontiers of human knowledge.

Do the politicians who put forward these ideas really believe them? Even in our own country we may well ask, what about William Shakespeare? Did he live in a world of economic security from the cradle to the grave? Did he have the advantage of the finest modern education? Indeed he did not, but he wrote the greatest English that has ever been set down. He did

not receive this type of education. He LAID DOWN THE STAND-
ARDS TO BE FOLLOWED LATER—how sadly have we followed
them. The best we can do is to keep on repeating Shakespeare's
wonderful English. None of us can write it any more. This is
true also of the achievements of the Greeks five hundred years
B.C. We have to go and see what they have done and we are
well content with what they have left—ruined as it is. We
cannot in any way emulate them.

Let our education then be of an individual nature. We are
never too old to commence learning. Education begins with a
keen observation so do not take someone else's word to be true
or the reasons given for any occurrence to be correct. Observe
for yourself and reason out your own explanation. If it is not
correct, you will still have begun to exercise your mind. In
time you will learn to observe accurately and make correct
deductions concerning your observations. This was the secret of
success of the forerunner of all true physicians—HIPPOCRATES.

Let us learn another lesson from the Greeks. "Nothing to
Excess". This is written over their temples—moderns interpret
this as meaning "do not get drunk" but it has a much wider
significance than this. It is a warning against over-specialization,
against pigeon-holing knowledge—to the Greek the all-rounder
was far better a man than the specialist and this applied to his
physical life as well as his mental existence. He would have
abhorred the modern version of the Olympic Games. To win in
the Sacred Grove of Olympia and to receive the olive crown of
victory, the athlete had to win many contests of varying skills—
in other words he had to be a good all-rounder, otherwise
Pindar would certainly not have written an ode to him.

To be a good all-rounder enables an individual to enjoy life
more fully and to live more completely. It enables life to be
carried on in complete harmony with the vibrations of the
inner and external world. THIS IS TRUE NATUROPATHY.

CHAPTER 4

PHYSICIAN HEAL THYSELF

This well-known quotation is worthy of our attention. Obviously the practitioner who can inspire the most confidence in his patient is the one who looks well himself; the one who obviously has vitality and is alert and observant. The man who in his own practical experience has in a personal sense practised the philosophy of Naturopathy is the one who can best show the patient the way back to health. Make sure your own life conforms to the tenets you hand to your patients and you will inspire them as an example. This will make it much easier for them to adopt and carry through the many changes in living which may be necessary for them in their efforts to regain their health.

The way back to health is often long, and a patient may need a great deal of encouragement with constant assurances of ultimate success. None can do this better than the practitioner who does in fact practise what he preaches. Nothing convinces like true sincerity, and true sincerity only comes of a genuine practice on the part of the preacher of the principles he teaches.

Division of the Cause of Disease

In Chapter 2 we outlined the basic causative factor of all disease as it affects the human organism. This basic cause may be sub-divided into three initial stages.

The first initial stage—this is lowered vitality which provides the preconditions for the accumulation of toxins in the cell structure. This is the beginning of the negative condition which produces disease. A mental attitude will lower vitality just as a physical cause, such as prolonged effort in one direction without a cycle of rest to conform to the body rhythm. Each cell while being in a sense a separate individual form of life—breathing, eating, drinking (eliminating and assimilating) as well as thinking—is at the same time interdependent on every other cell. Every cell depends on every other and disease ultimately commences with loss of harmony of vibration in a single cell.

The second initial stage—this is really the abnormal composition of blood and lymph. As soon as a cell or group of cells are ill, the rate of assimilation and elimination is changed, the nervous response is changed and thus whole groups of cells, namely the blood and lymph, are operating under adverse conditions and themselves become affected. The human organism, as we have seen, is made up biochemically of many substances, and it needs a variety of elements for its nourishment and continuance. Some are needed in greater quantities than others, while certain substances have to be present before the required nutrients can be absorbed and be useful. These latter substances are know as synergists.

Many of the substances that are required in small quantities are well-known and have achieved some popular acclaim in recent years. These are the so-called VITAMINS. This is really a misnomer as these so-called vitamins are chemical compounds which the body usually requires in very small amounts but whose presence is vital to health. Other substances needed in micro doses are the TRACE ELEMENTS. More of these substances when we deal with the practical application of the principles we are dealing with now.

It follows from this that if the cells and various organs of the body do not receive adequate supplies of these nutrients from the blood and lymph streams, all will not be well with the body and faulty functioning of the organism will result.

The third initial stage then is logically the accumulation of morbid matter, toxins and other waste products. These are encouraged to lodge in the cells and organs of the body, in time creating death and destruction to large groups of cells as the progress of the disease continues. This condition is seriously aggravated by the introduction of crude, suppressive allopathic drugs. These are toxins introduced into the organism needlessly.

Some of these such as arsenic, lead, etc. are cumulative and quite often are of such a nature that it is impossible for the body to eliminate them under any circumstances. This is, of course, why treatments involving the use of mercury, and other heavy metals are to be avoided at all costs if the patient is ever to get well again. Here the practitioner is very fortunate if the patient has come to him direct for naturopathic treatment before having run the gamut of orthodoxy first.

Secondary Causes of Disease

These are three kinds as follows :

1. Fevers, ulcerations, abscesses, inflammations and skin eruptions. These conditions are fertile soil for the multiplication of germs, bacteria and virus attacks and all are the end products of the three initial stages.
2. The miasms of Hahnemann (Psora, Sycosis, Syphilis) Tuberculosis, Cancer and all the other congenital taints with which the patient may have been born. We can also class the results of lead, mercurial, arsenical poisoning etc., under this heading.
3. All the different forms of insanity, nervous exhaustion, mechanical displacements of muscle structures, ligaments etc. subluxations (example of vertebrae), loss of self-control and hypersensitivity which can produce the same physical symptomology as poison by the heavy metals.

It may be thought at first sight that heredity disease is an initial cause rather than an end process. But a little reasoning will convince that this cannot be so. If the parents had adopted the correct procedure under Naturopathic Treatment, there would have been no taint in the child. The primary cause is therefore with the parents. It does not follow though that in these cases there is no cure. It is often possible to eradicate completely all hereditary taints and miasms in children and even adults, and true vital health can be obtained for the first time.

Immunity to Disease

With a balanced regimen, the human organism need not be a constant prey to every lurking germ or virus. Immunity is "built in" as it were. Germs there certainly are, as we argued before, which can attack the body. But these make no lasting impression on a healthy organism. They cannot continue to exist if the body is always capable of effectively fighting back and destroying them. A healthy body IS ALWAYS CAPABLE OF DOING JUST THIS.

Germs have become an obsession with allopathic practitioners. They are in reality of very secondary importance as we have so clearly shown. That is why the Naturopath is not so concerned with killing the germs to cure disease as in raising the body's vitality so that it can become healthy again and incidentally getting rid of the germs itself by creating the anti-bodies which make the continuance of the life of the germ impossible. Hence the futility of the powerful antiseptics, germicides, suppressive drugs and the rest of the negative methods employed by allopathic medicine today in its endless and ever failing task of killing germs. We know that as soon as some success has been reached in wiping out certain species of bacteria, a new resistant group is ever ready to take its place. It is an endless circle and a completely negative quest. Naturopathy has no part in this, we offer health by adherence to safe, sane and logical methods of treatment which, when properly and energetically applied, can scarcely fail. After all, germs are like man—adaptable—and they also have the will to live and to survive. If their environment is changed by drugs, in time they will learn how to live in the new environment. In fact, we do have a situation whereby some germs have learned to live with man causing him no harm, knowing instinctively that to kill their host is to end their own existence.

Cure

This follows the same logical laws as does the progress of disease, and here again we are at complete variance with the allopathic system of medicine. Colds, fevers, inflammations are suppressed. Mechanical defects are often provided with crutches in the shape of bindings, etc. Naturopathic treatment will support none of this. We must never suppress fevers or inflammatory conditions with drugs, or for that matter by any other means. These are the body's efforts to cure itself and they must be encouraged. These conditions, if properly treated, will follow an orderly course, leaving the patient very much better and fitter than before if, during the course of the condition, he does everything possible to facilitate it and encourage the Vital Force to do its work properly.

Very often a patient suffering from the chronic conditions of which we have written will find in a very short time that he is feeling very much worse than when he first came for treatment. This is where the importance of having the patient's cooperation comes in. The facts must be explained to him and he must be told what to expect in advance and not left to find himself suddenly experiencing distressing symptoms which in his ignorance can frighten him into discontinuing the treatment without further consultation with the practitioner. Correct naturopathic treatment will bring the chronic condition to the surface and the patient must be prepared for this. Acute symptoms may manifest themselves in the shape of fevers, skin eruptions etc. Headaches and internal turmoil will occur, and all these the patient must bear with fortitude, having been given confidence in advance by his practitioner. These of course are the HEALING CRISES of which we learned earlier.

Healing Crisis

The observant practitioner will make full use of the healing crisis and from it he will know just how much and just how long the Vital Force is capable of fighting to restore the patient's health. He will know from each healing crisis as it presents itself what new instructions to give the patient. The crisis itself is part of the reconstructive principle of the cure. It hastens the elimination of toxins and all the results of the disease processes from the system. It frees the cells, organs, blood, lymph etc., from the clogging effect of this accumulation and then the new-found freedom experienced as a result speeds up still further the elimination of impurities from the system while new, wholesome, constructive elements are brought to help rebuild and repair the damaged structures.

In this way, perhaps after the occurrence of several healing crises, the body will steadily re-establish that harmonious vibration within itself that is essential to health.

To produce a Healing Crisis, we may use, for instance, cold water baths to stimulate activity of the skin (Hydrotherapy). We may use herbal medicines, for example, alteratives, in the case of deep-seated miasms, or very high potency homoeopathic remedies which will effect and produce just the correct reaction from the Vital Force which we need for the particular case. In cases of mechanical defects of the body, we have physiotherapy and osteopathy as our main armaments.

The Healing Crisis, by no matter what means we bring it about, is the acute reaction of the Vital Force which immediately begins to bring about an improvement in the body. It always facilitates the elimination of the disease conditions, and although very often unpleasant while it lasts, can only have beneficial results. It is the opposite of the Disease Crisis. In the Disease Crisis the Vital Force is no longer powerful enough to cause the necessary reaction in the organism to produce elimination of the causative factors of the disease. In the Healing Crisis on the other hand, the Vital Force is doing its work and causing the body itself to react sharply to its disease condition by throwing off the toxins and instituting a regeneration of the whole organism.

The Principles for Which We Stand

We have dwelt at some length on the methods we employ in our treatments and some of the reasons why we employ them. We have given an outline of the philosophy of Naturopathy in the general sense and have provided in these first chapters something of the foundation on which, in future chapters, we shall elaborate with outline and details, practical application of the methods of which we now have an outline theoretical knowledge.

The reader will learn to use these methods according to the tenets we have propounded, and in co-ordinating the various aspects of treatment for the benefit of a particular patient, he may rest assured he is always doing the best possible under all circumstances and that no other system of medicine can offer such hope to suffering humanity as can Naturopathy under the guidance of a properly trained and well-informed exponent.

CHAPTER 5

MAN—THE MICROCOSM : MAN—THE MACROCOSM

We have seen how, in relative circumstances, man can be an infinity and is the macrocosm of his own internal forces. On the other hand, he is the microcosm in the universe which is external to him. We have seen that his position in both these spheres is interdependent. We also have a rough outline of the substances and forces which make up man, the macrocosm and we must now observe something of the surroundings in which man the microcosm finds himself. In order to do this, it is not a bad plan to adopt for the time being the terminology of the ancient alchemists.

Air—Water—Earth—Fire

These are termed the four great cardinal elements which support human life on this planet. They are usually put in the following order—Earth, Air, Fire and Water, but although life would be impossible without any one of these cardinal elements, they are here placed in what we consider their relative importance. It has been well said that man can only live a few minutes without air. He can live a somewhat longer time without water given the other three, and he can live even longer without food (Earth) while Fire (light and heat allied to all the other wave lengths) is the element which may be termed the common denominator or catalyst of the other three as it permeates the whole of man's surroundings. Certain reactions of the other three can also release Fire (energy). Man can also do this within himself and it is indeed this constant release of energy which makes life, as we know it, possible.

Rhythm

Our breathing has a definite rhythm even as have the tides of the earth, it affects the heart beat which in turn governs the rhythmic flow of blood throughout the human system. This breathing is governed either consciously or subconsciously by the psychic power manifesting through the Vital Force of each individual. This rhythm is duplicated in the wider field of the world outside by the influence of the moon. It is the influence of the moon which creates the tides and rhythms of the world. We can see from this how the ancients derived their word "lunatic". It was said that under certain circumstances the moon could influence men's minds directly and affect their psychic personality. The old alchemists were not so wrong in this inference and the word has only fallen into disrepute in very recent years with the advent of specialization in the mental field of therapeutics where the wood itself has been lost in the study of the individual trees.

Light

The moon in its turn depends on the sun (fire) for its position of influence in our solar system; and while the moon governs the night (the periods of psychic and mental activity), the sun rules the day (the period of physical action). In ancient times Apollo was worshipped as the God of Light (or the God of the Divine Radiance). This worship was of a principle and not an idol as the Christian Church has insisted. Apollo thus became the Patron of Man's Culture. He led man towards an appreciation of beauty. He was the supreme teacher of the Arts, Music, Literature, Architecture, Sculpture, as well as the exponent of physical perfection which men sought after in their exercises in the sunlight. His philosophy was positive and at the same time he was the God of Medicine. This is a significant point for it illustrated the fact that men appreciated the fact that health was obtained only by the all-round pursuit of the many activities of which Apollo was the God. It was later that his healing powers were delegated to his son, Aesculapius.

It is the Light and Heat coupled with a variety of other

lesser known vibrations and influences of the sun which pervade our earth and permit the reproductive and growth factors to manifest. Under its benign influence we are born, we develop, mature and ultimately decay. In the finite sense it is the influence of decay and change as well as of birth, growth and fulfilment.

Light also is the bridge by which we cross from the material physical world to the unseen world beyond. The rate of vibration of Light borders on the etheric and so to be in accord with the influence of Apollo is to take that path which leads to ultimate perfection of mind and body.

Earth

Even as the all-embracing light of the sun assists our human growth and maturity, so does it profoundly influence the growth of our Food. It is the action of the sunlight on the soil which in the laboratory of nature produces nutrients which are perfectly balanced for our assimilation. So perfectly is this system integrated that, if we follow the laws of healthful living in this way, we cannot help but be well and remain well through all the cycles of human evolution.

The Cardinal Elements

The careful appreciation of the influence of these Cardinal Elements impresses upon us the totality of man. This is yet another standpoint on which Naturopathy differs so widely from the orthodox accepted system of allopathic medicine.

Throughout the practice of Naturopathy, we must never be led to give over-importance to one or other of the branches of Natural Healing at the expense of the whole. Breathing and diet are, as we have seen, important to health, but one is not really more important than the other in the ultimate. The application of the principles of Hydrotherapy (water treatments), the use of Light and Heat or the employment of Osteopathy in the adjustment of some mechanical defect are equally important. One is no more important than the others. It is essential that we realize this, especially at the present time.

Many so-called naturopathic practitioners attach much more importance to the practice of Osteopathy than they do to any other form of natural treatment. This is because Osteopathy over recent years has become a vogue and is considered "fashionable" in certain circles of society.

Omnilateral Application

In doing this the practitioner has reduced himself and his ability to help his patients to the level of allopathic practice. This is the practice of specialization and giving the patient what in ignorance he thinks is good rather than what the practitioner should know in his greater wisdom as being the best for the patient. In fact, this is doing what so many naturopathic schools condemn the allopathic schools for doing—pandering to vested interests and carrying out certain treatments because of their commercial value rather than for the benefit of their patients. It is only by the omnilateral (many sided) application of the forces of healing that the patient can be cured. Osteopathy, dietetics, heat treatments, light treatments, etc., can become "gimmicks" when used in a unilateral way. They prove the inability of the practioner to appreciate the basic teachings of Naturopathy. They prove that such a practitioner is not a skilled Naturopath. In fact he could be in need of treatment himself.

Philosophy and Practice

We are now drawing to that stage in our study when we shall translate our philosophical concepts of Naturopathy into a practical system of healing. But if we are to practise with success either as practitioners or by putting this knowledge to practical use in our lives, we must never lose sight of the principles on which we act and always be in a position to reason out for ourselves a satisfactory explanation for what we do or what we are instructing a patient to do. If we can always do this, it will be easy to explain everything to our own satisfaction and to that of the patient, clearly and concisely.

Deep thought lies behind our action but our explanations must be simple and direct. It brings with it a directive force of the utmost value. It is the impetus which makes its practical application smooth, logical and ultimately successful.

Observation and Method

From the study of our philosophy we have been taught the immense importance of careful observation of the patient even if the patient is oneself. A meticulous catalogue must be recorded of all the signs and symptoms observed and investigated.

Never stint time on this. Always record a full history including details of employment, social background, likes, dislikes and everything and anything which can be of any possible importance in arriving at an understanding of the underlying causes of the condition presented for treatment.

Diagnosis

This evaluation we call diagnosis and it will be dealt with fully in a practical sense in the following chapters. Every piece of evidence you can elicit about the disease and every little detail you can collect in respect of the case will help in arriving at as accurate a picture as possible and be of immense assistance in plotting the course the disease will take during care and treatment.

Prognosis

The art of foretelling the course the disease will take is known as prognosis, and only by making a really accurate diagnosis in the first place can you in turn make a good prognosis. On this will depend all the information and instructions you are able to give the patient. The art of doing this will be explained in the chapters dealing with the practical application of Naturopathy.

Pathology

The morbid changes which take place and come under the heading of Secondary Causes of Disease (Chapter 4) are called pathological. The second classification of our secondary causes in particular deals with pathological changes which take place in the tissues and organs of the body. Careful attention has to be given to these and special assistance is required so that the body can eliminate the toxins as quickly as possible. We deal with pathology also in a practical way in later chapters.

Treatment

This will always be worked out bearing in mind the patient's present condition. You will always use the greatest number of means possible to restore health. Never suppress the symptoms. The practitioner never cures the patient. The patient will be assisted to cure himself.

The many and varied means at our disposal for the practical application of our already stated philosophy now follow in the practical section of this book.

In addition to dealing with diagnosis, prognosis and pathology, concrete details will be given of the various treatments carried out in all the different spheres of influence. These will include Hydrotherapy, Dietetics, Vitaminotherapy, the famous Schroth Cure, Fasting, Physiotherapy and Electrotherapy. In addition, deficiency diseases as well as some of the effects of excesses of different kinds will be covered.

PART 2

DIETETICS

CHAPTER 6

FOOD REFORM

Correct diet, as we have already seen, is one of the great cornerstones of Naturopathic Practice. It is essential, therefore, that any would-be practitioner must have a very sound knowledge of food values and the correct application of various foodstuffs in a particular combination suitable to the treatment of individual disease conditions. "Individual disease conditions" because, although in many cases group symptomologies are observed which present a rather similar picture in different patients and lead to the use of general names for "diseases", THEY ARE ALWAYS INDIVIDUAL DISEASE CONDITIONS and a very different diet or combination of foodstuffs may be required in the case of one patient from that of another offering a very similar set of symptoms. This is where an appreciation of other than the purely physical factors of the case may be required. The educational background may be different, occupation may be different, living conditions generally may be different, economic resources may vary and in fact all these physical differences may be in addition to differences in mental and spiritual outlook as well as differences in psychic development. For these and many other reasons no two patients may be treated alike and the naming of groups of similar symptoms as one disease or another is at best a very vague generalization.

Reforming the diet must be done with due regard to these

indications in addition to the availability of the foodstuffs indicated—the season of the year during which treatment is carried out and the ability of the patient to follow correctly the instructions given. Fortunately today very few areas with any density of population are without a good Health Food Store service and more and more retailers are catering for the ever increasing demand for naturally grown and fertilized vegetables, fruits and other food products, all of which makes the task of the Naturopath that much more simple in this respect. In the case of meat products also it is now possible to obtain fresh meat from animals which have lived healthy natural lives and eggs from hens which have had "to scratch for a living" (free range). There are today Health Food Stores which combine the sale of the usually accepted "Health Foods" with that of naturally composted vegetables, cereals and their products as well as naturally reared and fed meat, etc. This is a great step forward and proves conclusively that more and more people are rebelling against the inhumanly cruel systems of intensive breeding and feeding of animals for the sake of ever larger profits for the producers concerned.

The Function of Food

The function of food is twofold. First it must supply energy to the body and make this available. This energy can manifest in two ways. It can take the form of heat when the body temperature is higher than that of its surroundings. This means that if you are in a cold place you will need a supply of energy from your food in order to be able to maintain your normal body temperature. Secondly you need energy so that you can move about, so that your organs can function. Movement of any kind of the body requires energy and this it obtains by absorbing food and converting it into energy.

The second function of food is to supply the cells and tissues with fresh material to replace those worn and wasted. This wearing or wasting can be either through over-exercise when the body becomes depleted until fresh supplies of tissue building material are made available, or following disease when the

Vital Force has been stimulated to use up reserves and make inroads into what is required immediately for minute to minute living.

In the case of women in pregnancy, when the diet is inadequate the supply of fresh material will be sadly lacking and the mother will in some measure suffer at the expense of the unborn child. Excessive fasting will also deplete the organism but of this we shall have much more to say when we are actually dealing with fasts as therapeutic agents.

Food Classification

In recent years the advent of new discoveries of food factors, micro nutrients etc., even the allopathic conception of food values has undergone a change and has come more in line with the ideas put forward by Naturopathy over many decades. Before going carefully into these, we shall consider food classification from the old established system as this will help us fully to understand nutrition in relation to disease and cure, when we are dealing with diet as a treatment of various kinds of disease.

Proteins—Fats—Carbohydrates

These are the main classes of food which make up human nutrition. In order to use the food, the body first breaks it down by the process of digestion—this is known as CATABOLISM. Having, as it were, provided itself with the raw materials, the body then uses these basic substances to build up the many and complex substances of living tissue. This process is known as ANABOLISM. The whole work of breaking down and building up which is constantly going on in the human body is known as METABOLISM. This does not only happen in man but is carried on throughout nature. For example, for vegetation to grow, many chemical compounds are broken down and then used again and built into the tissues of growing plants from the soil. In the case of animals, the process is much the same as in man.

Proteins

These we may call the body builders. They are vital factors in growth, repair and replacement. Without protein life cannot exist. Age requires more protein than youth. Nitrogen is the main factor and one of the distinguishing characteristics of proteins. They also contain several other elements such as Hydrogen, Sulphur, Carbon, Oxygen and Phosphorus. All are important, but Nitrogen is found in every protein, all the other elements are not.

The main point to remember is that even in deep sleep our heart and lungs are using up proteins. In using them, they are broken down and excreted. They cannot be used again. This means that there is a continuous loss of nitrogenous matter and it is absolutely necessary in consequence that any diet should contain an adequate amount of proteins to replace this constant loss.

A great Greek philosopher many centuries B.C. said "Life is Movement". This is absolutely true, for without movement there can be no life and we must remember that without proteins there can be no movement (life). The following are a few examples of proteins :

Casein—in milk
Albumen—in egg white
Myosin—in lean meat
Globutin—in egg yoke
Fibrin—in clotted blood
Gluten—in wheat

It is important to know that amino-acids are the precursors of proteins. These are compounds which the body uses in the building up part of metabolism (anabolism). Most of these amino-acids MUST be provided by food as the body cannot synthesize these for itself or at least only a few of them.

Every cell, as we shall see in later studies, consists of proto-plasm and protoplasm itself holds in suspension, as it were, a balanced mixture of all the nutrients required for life. By far the most important of these is protein. The finest proteins for human assimilation are undoubtedly derived from eating animal tissue. Meat, fish, eggs and cheese are first-class proteins. Sweet fruits, nuts and pulses are known as second-class proteins.

Nitrogen Loss

If the body is inadequately supplied with proteins, the loss of nitrogen from the body will be greater than that taken in by food. This can have quite a serious effect and in fact can result in premature ageing. For instance, the hair and finger nails are in reality true excreta of the body. They consist of almost pure proteins. If the body is deprived of these vital materials, it will in time become unable to maintain the steady strength of this excreta, with the result that the hair and finger nails will rapidly deteriorate in appearance with results which can be seen around us every day.

Unfortunately, all too little is known about proteins themselves, despite a great deal of research by biochemists, and until recent years the proteins have tended to be neglected in favour of a study of vitamins, while previously carbohydrates and fats held the limelight.

Amino-Acids

Although there is still a great deal to learn about proteins, we do know much more about the precursors of proteins, which we call amino-acids. These are the next stage in complexity from the Elements themselves which we have already listed. From the protoplasm, which contains a balanced mixture of all three of the food classes and is therefore the most complex, we descend via proteins—metaproteins, proteoses-peptones-poly-peptides to amino acids. There are between twenty and thirty known amino-acids and there could be many more. These combine together in a variety of ways to form proteins and have many things in common with the other two main classes of food (fats and carbohydrates) while at the same time having many entirely unique features. This illustrates their supreme importance.

These facts alone should now make the reader conscious of

the importance of proteins in the diet and no diet can be balanced without the inclusion of proteins.

Fats and Carbohydrates

Carbohydrates are the starches and sugars, and with the fats they are first and foremost the fuels of the body, but do not forget that proteins also provide energy and are as good in this respect as carbohydrates. Fats on the other hand are the best fuel as they give out more heat per unit of weight than do either the proteins or the carbohydrates. Life can be supported on a fat free diet or a diet free of carbohydrates, but it cannot be supported without proteins.

Fats and Obesity

It is quite possible that for economic reasons the diet of the large majority contains a preponderance of carbohydrates with the result that many people become overweight and suffer from obesity. There are also types who do not actually overeat starches and sugars but who still suffer from this distressing condition. In other words, there are types who for metabolic reasons cannot make full use of these fuels. These people can usually make do very well with the fats, and if the diet is adjusted to increase the fat and protein intake and to cut the starches and sugars down to a minimum, they will immediately begin to reduce weight. Here is a case of eating fat to get rid of fat. It is only in the tropical and sub-tropical climates where a greatly reduced carbohydrate diet may become intolerable. In the polar regions of the earth men live very well on an almost pure protein and fat diet.

Cane Sugar

Cane sugar or sucrose is the purest form of carbohydrate, and glucose is the simplest form of carbohydrate. All carbohydrates taken in the form of food are broken down into glucose before being circulated in the blood to the muscles to be burnt up as heat or used to maintain body heat. Two kinds of energy are produced by either proteins, carbohydrates or fats which are used as fuels and ultimately broken down to be used as energy. The energy used for producing movement in the body is known as KINETIC ENERGY. That for maintaining body temperature is called THERMAL ENERGY.

Under Proteins we stated that they were the most complex while the amino-acids were the most simple of this type of food. Here Glucose is the simplest form of carbohydrate but we have two substances which tie as being the most complex forms. These are cellulose and starch. Glucose is only one of the simplest forms of monosugars, but is enough for our purpose.

Cellulose

Cellulose can be broken down in the laboratory to the simple sugars, but the digestion of man is incapable of doing this and therefore cellulose acts as a roughage. Cellulose is the main constituent of the walls of the cells of vegetables.

Hydrolysis and Condensation

When carbohydrates are broken down, the term used for the process is Hydrolysis, and when they are made complex by combining them together the process is known as Condensation, or in the body as we have said before—anabolism and catabolism.

When starch is broken down in the body (hydrolysis) there are present certain substances which speed up or help to promote this process. These substances are called enzymes or ferments and the action they produce is one of catalysis.

Many forms of bacteria produce enzymes or ferments and in the intestinal tract of man are to be found many benign forms of bacteria which produce enzymes which are essential for the utilization of our food.

Fats and Oils

For our purpose there is one group of oils only that come under the heading of FATS as body fuels. These are the fatty oils. There are in fact two other kinds of oil :

1. Mineral oils, such as paraffin, petroleum, etc., and

2. The essential oils extracted from fruits and flowers.

Neither of these kinds of oil provide fuel for the body and little is known of the effect of the essential oils although many are reputed to have valuable therapeutic properties which can be used in conjunction with herbal medicines. The Mineral Oils are distinct in that they consist only of hydrogen and carbon and consequently are called hydro-carbons. Before passing from these however it is interesting to note that at least one hydrocarbon does play a very valuable role in human metabolism. This hydrocarbon is called CAROTENE and is the precursor of Vitamin "A" but this will be dealt with fully under Vitaminotherapy.

The oxygen content of the fats and fatty oils is much lower than in carbohydrates. They all have one thing in common— they are decomposed by alkalis. This is known as being saponifiable. In other words, they will produce a soap and glycerine (an alcohol).

In the body it would appear that fats and fatty oils are broken down in the intestines to form glycerine and fatty acid salts. But a great deal has still to be learned in this direction. The pancreas in addition to the intestines, secretes lipases which are enzymes assisting the breakdown of fats in the same way as in the laboratory an alkali would be used.

Fats and Vitamins

It is probably much more true to say that the lipases (enzymes) permit only a certain amount of breakdown of the fats in the intestines producing enough soap to combine with the bile salts to form a fine emulsion which will then pass through intestinal cells via the capillaries into the blood and the lymph systems.

There is still much research work to be done on the subject of fats and the soluble and insoluble fatty acids. These products are not simply body fuels as are the carbohydrates, for they also contain the oil soluble vitamins which are another essential part of our nutrition and which will be dealt with separately.

The Balanced Diet

We have now dealt with the three groups of foods and from what we have learnt we should know that it is essential to have some of all three classes of food to form a balanced diet. We should know also that a fat and protein diet will produce more energy than a protein carbohydrate diet and can in fact be used to reduce weight as less of the fats are needed to produce the same amount of energy as starch.

All these classes of foods contain four elements occurring in organic (organized) combination, viz. carbon, hydrogen, oxygen and nitrogen. In addition, protein contains sulphur and phosphorus in organic form.

Foods also contain a residue ash of combustion and it is in this we find the mineral elements. 95 per cent of our food is made up of the three classes we have discussed, while the remaining 5 per cent contains the vitamins, trace elements, mineral elements, etc. These, although occupying such a small proportion of the total, are of vital importance in maintaining health.

CHAPTER 7

MINERALS

Mr. Five Per Cent

At the end of the last chapter we stated that after the three classes of food with which we have already dealt, there is 5 per cent which consists of the major mineral elements and the trace elements, vitamins, etc. This 5 per cent is a most important part of our nutrition and it can be subdivided into two parts. That part which will occupy us now—the main mineral elements and a part we shall deal with later—the trace elements, vitamins, filtrate factors, etc.

The Principal Elements

These are:

POTASSIUM (K)	SODIUM (Na)	CALCIUM (Ca)
MAGNESIUM (Mg)	IRON (Fe)	PHOSPHORUS (P)
SULPHUR (S)	SILICON (Si)	CHLORINE (Cl)

Potassium

Potassium is an essential ingredient of blood corpuscles. It is said to be one of the elements which helps to preserve youth, and a serious deficiency will result in early death. There is a theory that a deficiency of potassium will cause cancer and allied conditions. Potassium is also in the brain and nerve cells and in cases of deficiency it is from the brain and nerve cells that the body will obtain its potassium LAST OF ALL. This gives rise to the theory that the brain and nerve fibres suffer least of all from cancerous conditions as the body strives with might and main to preserve the potassium content here as long as possible.

Sodium

This element is closely akin to potassium. They are, it can be said, so closely allied that in certain circumstances one can be substituted for the other, but when this occurs in the case of potassium deficiency, it hastens old age and death. Sodium, as we all know, is the metal which forms the salt sodium chloride, and this salt is everywhere around us as well as in the body fluids. The body is richer in sodium than in any other metal. Chlorine has an important role in the body in maintaining these two metals SODIUM and POTASSIUM as CHLORIDES. The part played by sodium chloride is perhaps mainly physiological in that it maintains OSMOTIC pressure. This is the balance of pressure inside and outside the walls of blood vessels, lymph, etc. The salt solution is able to pass from that on the stronger side to that on the weaker and so maintain the balance.

Calcium

This element occurs mainly in oxide form in bones and teeth and is essential to proper growth and development. Lime Phosphate and carbonate salts containing the elements carbon, oxygen and phosphorus show how these combine for this purpose. From this we again see how important it is for the protein in our daily diet to be adequate since it makes these elements available.

Phosphorus

In the same way as Sodium and Potassium are very closely akin so are CALCIUM and PHOSPHORUS. They occur in combination as phosphates and the one is of no use without the other. Unlike the case of Sodium and Potassium they will not replace each other. They are both essential and are necessary in the blood stream. Any deficiency of these phosphates will most certainly lead to illness and death. For their adequate use, they require in addition VITAMIN "D" which we shall deal with later. Three-quarters of a gramme are needed daily.

Magnesium

This important element is also closely related to Calcium and

Phosphorus and together they form a sort of trinity of elements. It is also significant that magnesium nearly always occurs with calcium and phosphorus in our food stuffs. It is essential food for the nervous system and the brain as magnesium phosphate.

Other elements closely associated with these three are arsenic, strontium and barium, and may be necessary as traces. We know very little about this but is it now known that arsenic in minute traces does play some part in human metabolism.

Iron

Most of us know that iron is essential for good quality blood. It is in fact the principal component of haemoglobin (a protein) which carries the oxygen in the blood from the lungs to all parts of the body. As most of us know, when this part of the chemistry of the body breaks down, we have conditions of anaemia—another sound reason for adequate protein supplies in the diet. It is also said that traces of arsenic and cobalt are necessary as they act as fixatives or synergists of iron in the blood. Green vegetables form our best supply of iron and it is well to remember this in practice for various forms of nutritional anaemia are widespread among all age groups and this can lead to forms of arthritis later in life if not properly treated. The old empirical iron remedies are useless for this purpose but herbal medicines are a wonderful adjunct to good treatment of these conditions.

Sulphur

This is another element necessary for the proper function of the nerves. It acts in many ways and may even have a germicidal effect in the organism. It occurs in nearly all the proteins and is indispensable in our nutrition. Yet another reason for an adequate intake of daily proteins.

Silicon

We have placed this under the heading of Principal Elements but it does in fact also belong to the trace elements. Very little is yet known of the true value of silicon in the metabolism. We know that it promotes suppuration and elimination of toxic waste and is required also for healthy hair, bones, teeth, etc., and is another of those elements which are supposed to be linked with the preservation of youth by maintaining the integrity of human tissues. There is more to say on this as a trace element in Chapter 8.

Chlorine

This, as we have seen, helps and is an important fact in holding potassium and sodium in solution in the body fluids. Research in the years to come may have a great deal more to say about this element. We all know from our schooldays chemistry that it does in fact form a trinity of gases with Bromine and Iodine and it is significant that Iodine is a very important constituent of the human body. It helps to form the hormone secreted by the thyroid gland (Thyroxine).

We have now covered the main elements which make up part of the remaining 5 per cent after the 95 per cent represented by the first three main classes of food which we have dealt with.

We have discovered some of the work these elements do in the body and in what way they are used in the metabolic processes.

We shall now repeat the list of elements, giving some of the results and therapeutic uses so as to form a guide as to what to expect in certain conditions and what foods or remedies to prescribe for overcoming deficiencies of one or the other.

Therapeutic Uses

POTASSIUM : is required for the generation of electric forces in the body. It provides suppleness and flexibility to muscles, joints and arteries. It will build up flesh and preserve youth and healthy activity.

SODIUM : As we have said, being found in all the body fluids, it is also present in the gastric juices and promotes digestion. It helps in the elimination of uric acid and other waste products from the system.

CALCIUM : Most vital for the very young and growing. Useful in all bone diseases. It assists in toning up the muscles and lack of it will bring about brittle bones, tooth decay and lassitude.

MAGNESIUM: Of great value in getting rid of all kinds of toxins from the body. One of the scavenger elements as well as being a tonic for the brain and nerves in the form of magnesium phosphate.

PHOSPHORUS: The great brain and nerve stimulator, as well as helping in the repair of bone structures when broken and in maintaining the organism free from bacteriacidal attack, especially the lungs (the tubercle bacillus is destroyed by phosphoric acid secreted in healthy lungs).

SULPHUR: This is valuable as a remedy for rheumatism, gout and many skin disorders. As has already been said, it is a laxative though not one to be used with indiscretion. It combines again to produce valuable disinfectants in the organism.

SILICON: Necessary in cases of weak muscle structure, tendons and ligaments in particular. It absorbs poisons in the system and helps in their excretion.

CHLORINE: Has a predilection for the alimentary tract and is useful in disorders of the stomach and liver.

IRON: This is the great body strengthener and combines in the red blood corpuscles to carry oxygen to all parts of the body. It is a valuable tonic for many run down conditions. A minimum of 11 milligrams per day are required.

In working out a personal diet, always find out first which nutrients you require to prescribe in the greatest abundance and then compose the diet bearing in mind the foods which contain a preponderance of what you require. If you wish to prescribe iron to correct a deficiency, then think in terms of watercress, lettuce and dandelion leaves, etc. If it is phosphorus that is required, then apples, wheat, lemons and more particularly kale, parsley and brussels sprouts. Sodium can be obtained from strawberries, tomatoes and leeks. The foods richest in silicon are sprouts, dandelion and cauliflower. For potassium deficiency prescribe foods like peaches, apricots and lemons, tomatoes, lettuce and celery. The calcium foods are too well known to mention here. Celery and tomatoes are also among the richest food sources of chlorine as is butter.

CHAPTER 8

THE TRACE ELEMENTS

It is impossible to deal exhaustively with the subject of the trace elements, their role in human health and their importance in the soil for the growing of the foodstuffs we eat. This is because our knowledge of the subject is still in its early stages and not because it is unimportant to our study. There is still much research work to be done in this field. We know, however, even at this stage that the trace elements are an extremely important aspect of human nutrition and they can be intelligently used in helping to combat disease and promote health.

Perhaps the most important Element which is also a trace element in the human organism is SILICON and this we shall deal with last and at length. Some of the other more important trace elements are :

Copper

We mentioned the disease anaemia earlier and stated that iron alone was not enough to cure nutritional anaemia. It is the presence of a trace element such as copper which makes the assimilation of copper by the body cell structure possible. The prescription of large doses of crude iron salts which was the vogue in Victorian times was extremely harmful as these salts leeched from the system the body's natural iron and only aggravated the condition in the long term. We now know that we must combine copper or perhaps a minute trace of arsenic with such treatment in order to obtain a lasting result, and how much better to prescribe food which has these essential nutrients in a properly balanced form. About two milligrams of copper are needed each day by the average individual.

Manganese

This trace element has a role somewhat similar to copper and in addition is associated with the reproductive system. It can offer help in cases of impotence in some obscure way not fully known.

Cobalt

Essential in small quantities, it has, in recent years, been thought to play a part in preventing the formation of dangerous acids in the system which lead to the very prevalent rheumatic complaints. It is also said to help in providing immunity to certain diseases, but very little indeed can be said definitely of this as yet. Its deficiency in British soil has also been put forward as a reason for the very high incidence of disseminated sclerosis in this country. This in these days of imports of many greater varieties of foods is less easy to define. It forms a part of the molecular structure of Vitamin B.12 and is further proof of the essential part played by this element in the prevention of anaemia and the rheumatic diseases.

Chromium

Vanadium, zinc, boron and tin are other important trace elements. Excess chrome in the system thought by some to be the result of the use of stainless steel cooking utensils is said to produce cancer and thrombosis while the use of vanadium in such cases was recently said by American researchers to antidote this. There is certainly a strong case against the use of stainless steel for cooking. Zinc is necessary for the maintenance of muscular control in the body and may be linked with the Vitamin B.6 in this respect. Boron is one of the trace elements of which no one is liable to be deficient and as age advances so does our store of zinc in the body. Tin is essential for the assimilation of silica and plays an important role in the body in this respect.

Silica (to preserve youth)

From the beginning of time the molten mass deep in the heart of our earth has been working away and always throwing upwards the substances which make up the solid crust we see around us in the form of mountains, meadows, and cliffs, covering which is a layer of soil. It is the gradual decomposition and powdering down or weathering of the rock formations of the mountains and cliffs over many thousands of years which produce the fertile soil which in turn is the medium of growth for our foodstuffs. This is nature's vast laboratory at work on its endless task of involution and evolution.

From the rough hard texture of granite and sandstone, marble and basalt is gently distilled the healing properties of our herbal remedies. The potassium, sodium and calcium with magnesium, iron and phosphorus are thus organized to our human needs and of all these by far the most abundant is silica —consider the sands of the sea shore. Nature is the Great Homoeopath—triturating and attenuating from time was until time is and will doubtless go on with this endless task in all the time that is to be. It is this constant grinding which alone can make all the important elements of human nutrition readily assimiliable. The triturated products of the soil are fired by the sun in the presence of the air to produce the plants on which we complex humans can live and from which in turn we derive our essential nutrition.

Silica, with which we are presently concerned, is derived from the element silicon and is the most important substance in the maintenance of tissue integrity in the human body. It is essential for the continued strength of all the connective tissues, such as ligaments, muscles, and bone structure. At the same time it plays a most important role in metabolism by promoting suppuration and the elimination of toxic waste from the system. Without it our bones would become brittle, our skin would lose its elasticity and youthful freshness, our teeth will rot and our hair become lifeless and fall out.

Surely then, this is one of the most important factors in the preservation of our youth. The first visible signs of age are falling and brittle hair with sagging skin and loss of muscular strength while, in old age come the brittle bones so prone to fracture—all because this vital silica is deficient and has most probably been deficient throughout life, so that nature in her human laboratory has had to make do with "second best" and build into our body tissues second-rate products in order to keep us going for as long as possible without breakdown. Nature will always strive for the best under any conditions, but when the best is not available second best has to do, which, in the end, leads to breakdown and disease in our human terms. Why is this? Why does nature so often have to make do with second best? The reason can always be found in the individual diet.

Just as it takes nature many thousands of years of continuous work to prepare and make substances available as perfect human nutrition, so in the individual human case it is only proper and complete nutrition through all the years of life which will provide our health and strength for the complete period of our life span.

Silica—an aid to youth it most certainly is—but it is not a wonder food which, if taken in a special diet for a few weeks, will eradicate the ravages of all the years of deficiency. Nature does not and will not work that way. If we are wise throughout our lives and always make sure our diet has had adequate amount of vital substances like silica we shall be rewarded with continued health and strength and the maintenance of our youthful looks and figure far on into old age. We will avoid the ravages of time as seen in those foolish people who place the satisfaction of palate before the nutritional needs of the body.

Failing sight is another sign of early old age and cataract is caused by silica deficiency. The eye muscles themselves will lose their elasticity thus restricting our powers of focus. In fact, silica is an essential constituent of all the connective tissues, fibres and the skin. Without it bones become brittle, muscles become slack and weak, ligaments which bind our joints together become loose and the skin wrinkles and sags—a sorry tale of "sans teeth, sans hair, sans eyes, sans everything".

How to prevent this terrible consequence of silica deficiency and is it too late? It is never too late, though, naturally, from what has already been stated the later it is left the less good will be the long-term results, and as to how, this is two-fold.

1. By the immediate adoption of a diet which will not only provide adequate supplies of silica, but all the other vital elements as well.

2. By trying to make up for lost time by supplementing the diet with specially manufactured forms of silica which, by careful compounding and trituration over long periods is made easily assimilable and readily absorbed into the tissues where it is so urgently needed.

Herbal Sources

It is well known among herbalists that Comfrey is an ideal remedy for fractures BUT, unfortunately, this is all too often used in the empirical sense and not because the reason for its efficacy is known. The fact is that Comfrey is a rich vegetable supply of silica. So is lung wort, which is why it is so useful in diseases of the pulmonary system, where there is a weakening of the connective and supporting tissues of the lungs. Hound's tongue and nettles are also rich sources of supply, while perhaps best of all is the horse-tail, which contains a high percentage of soluble silicic acid. Borage is also a herbal supplier of silica.

Food Supplement

Silica can be obtained in highly triturated biochemic form as cellules to be dissolved on the tongue and in this way is a valuable dietary supplement.

Food Sources

Sprouts, dandelions and cauliflower are the richest in silica and these foods should form a basic and constant part of the diet, especially in older people.

In conclusion, it should also be mentioned that silica is anti-cancerous and can be used therapeutically in all cases when suppuration is to be encouraged. Massive doses will avoid surgery in cases of abscess. It will help in the expulsion of foreign bodies from the tissues, it will preserve your eyesight and it can be

used with great advantage for the treatment of asthma (lungwort), epilepsy, rheumatism (comfrey) and, in fact, in all
diseases in which the connective and elastic tissues of the body
are affected. To preserve YOUR youth and vitality make sure that
your daily diet is rich in silica—it will completely replace the
need of drugs such as penicillin, etc.—and there are only good
side-effects.

The Vitamins

The last but not least important of our MR. FIVE PER CENT
are the vitamins. They are extremely complex substances in
many cases, and it is quite possible that there are still many
undiscovered vitamins. It is certain that however many undiscovered vitamins there may be, they do in fact already exist
in WHOLE FRESH NATURAL FOODS or the body is able from
other materials to synthetize its own.

Vitamins are organic substances which are found in animal
or vegetable tissues and are essential for the proper growth,
development and wellbeing of man. Like the mineral elements
and the trace elements, they do not provide energy, and are not
the building materials of the body. Without their presence, however, the generation of energy and the regulation of metabolism
would not be possible. They are required usually only in small
quantities daily to be completely effective, and indeed as we shall
see, too large doses of some vitamins can have a toxic effect.

Although Vitamins have been known for many years, some
of them for a much longer time than others, many of them
had not been actually isolated as definite compounds, and so
the idea was evolved of labelling them with letters of the alpha-
bet. This, in some cases, has led to confusion as have the names
given them, as these are sometimes different in America than
they are in this country. Others known for some time and
thought to have certain effects in the body have had their therapeutic uses changed in the light of recent research and more
up-to-date knowledge.

It is not necessary to go deeply into the chemistry of vitamins
for our purpose or to give a long historical account of their

discovery. There are many very good text books to be had on this subject alone and the reader has a wide choice if he wishes to make a special study of the subject of vitamins. Our main object is to present them here within the context of Naturopathic Practice and for this purpose we give their main uses and some guide as to individual human requirements under normal health conditions. In this way the reader will be able to use his knowledge of them in relation to the prescribing of specialized diets, etc.

Two Vitamin Categories

Vitamins are usually divided into two classes—the FAT SOLUBLE and the WATER SOLUBLE. As a general rule the fat soluble vitamins are better able to be stored in the body than are the water soluble variety as they are usually stored in organs like the liver. One fat soluble vitamin "D" can be manufactured by the body under the best conditions of living. These fat soluble vitamins, being more easily stored in the body, are the most liable to have toxic effects when taking in too great doses over long periods of time.

The Oil Soluble Vitamins

Vitamin "A"—In Chapter 6 we studied fats and how, with the assistance of lipases, they were broken down in the body to soap, but there is a fraction of unsaponifiable material in fish liver oils which contains Vitamin "A". This substance is very closely associated with the vegetable CAROTENE (the pro vitamin "A"). Vitamin "A" is stored principally in the liver, which can hold quantities for use in cases of temporary lack in the diet. Deficiency brings about degeneration and hardening of the skin cells, notably in the epithelium of the conjunctive of the nasal and respiratory passages as well as of the bladder and genital organs. Deficiency also weakens resistance to disease of the infectious type and interferes with the formation of teeth enamel. Early signs of this deficiency result in "night blindness" as the visual purple of the retina is partly composed of Vitamin "A".

Vitamin "A" is useful in the form of ointments for the treatment of burns, ulcers and senile skin conditions as well as for respiratory infections. It must be remembered that during pregnancy larger intakes of it are essential for the wellbeing of the mother and also during lactation. Vitamin "A" was only discovered as a separate substance from Vitamin "D" in the early 1920's.

The average daily requirements are said to be between four and six thousand international units for adults and between one and two thousand for children, but very much larger quantities can be tolerated without any toxic effects of any kind. In prescribing concentrated doses of this vitamin, it is advisable to give the patient periods of rest between courses.

Vitamin "D"—This is also a fat soluble vitamin and occurs in nature closely associated with Vitamin "A". It is perhaps the only vitamin that the human body can manufacture for itself by the effect of sunlight on the skin. It is known as the anti-rhacitic factor as it was discovered as being necessary for the prevention and cure of rickets in children around the year 1890, when this disease was first associated with lack of sunlight. It is essential to the calcium-phosphorus metabolism of the body and a lack of it will cause brittle bones that fracture easily. In other words, it is an essential factor in the growth of healthy bones and therefore of vital necessity to children in the formative years.

It has many uses in practice and cases of arthritis have been known to benefit from a diet supplemented with large doses. Hay fever, and asthma are other conditions which have benefited, also psoriasis, eczema and acne. For psoriasis and asthma, massive doses are required, in the region of 300,000–400,000 International Units. However, it can be said that this treatment on its own is not very successful and has somewhat declined in popularity in recent years.

It is possible to prescribe overdoses of Vitamin "D" when there is a toxic result in the organism, but it is highly unlikely that this can happen under ordinary circumstances. Anything over 10,000 I.U. per lb. of body weight would be considered dangerous.

The average daily requirements would appear to be between 500 and 600 I.U. for adults and between 600 and 700 I.U. for children. Rather more is required for children growing up in the smoke laden atmospheres of the cities where the ultra violet content of sunlight is absorbed before it can reach the skin. This would also apply to the northern latitudes where so much of the year is spent under winter conditions and with little or no sunlight.

VITAMINS "A" and "D", as we have stated, nearly always occur together in nature and if the right foods are prescribed which are rich in the one, then it can be taken for granted that the other will be there in sufficient quantity also.

Vitamin "E"—This was not isolated as alphatocopherol until 1938, and is generally known as the reproductive vitamin, although little is known so far as to its exact role in metabolism. Deficiency in the male over a long period can lead to degenerative changes in the epithelium of the testis with sterility which cannot be afterwards cured. In fact degenerative changes can occur in all tissues. It is known as the anti-sterility vitamin but today it is known not to play such a large part in this as was thought when it was first discovered. Like "A" and "D" it is fat soluble. It occurs mainly in seed foods, peanuts, lettuce, etc., and is essential for the nutrition of the nervous and muscular systems.

In practice it is used for cardiovascular disease with some success, but massive doses are needed in these conditions. It has not been found as successful as was supposed in the treatment of abortion or of impotence, although some degree of success in some cases has been observed. It certainly has properties rather like Vitamin "A" in that it seems in some measure to preserve firmness and youthfulness of tissue. The average daily requirements of this vitamin are not really known but something in the region of 10 mg are required and considerably more during pregnancy—about 2 grams per day.

Vitamin "K"—This is not really one substance at all but a

group of substances which occur mainly in green plants—alfalfa and lettuce seem to be the best sources of supply. Another oil soluble vitamin, very little is known of this group of substances at the present time except that they are essential for the formation of prothrombin and lack of it prolongs clotting time of the blood and causes liability to haemorrhage.

A daily human requirement has not been accurately given so far. Foods containing this vitamin or groups of substances are useful in cases where there is a congenital tendency to haemorrhage.

This concludes our survey of the oil soluble vitamins and in the next chapter we shall deal with the far more numerous water soluble ones and some of the filtrate factors.

CHAPTER 9

THE WATER SOLUBLE VITAMINS

Vitamin "B₁" and "B₂" Complex

Ancurine hydrochloride (Thiamin) is the chemical name given to "B₁". It is found throughout the body and is stored to a small extent in the liver, heart and kidneys and is found in the brain and nerve cells as well as muscles, lungs, spleen and blood. It is known as the anti-neuritic vitamin as long-term deficiency brings about pathological changes in the nerve fibres with all the symptoms of neuritis. Polyneuritis and Beri-Beri are the results of serious chronic deficiency.

The presence of aneurine is essential for the proper oxydation of carbohydrates, and without it the tissues are unable to take up the oxygen required, thus affecting respiration and causing damage to the organs mentioned above.

We can obtain this vitamin from animal liver, oats, wheat and other cereals, bananas and egg yolk. The average daily requirement is about 3 mg. It is known as being thermo-labile, that is, it is affected and destroyed by moist heat, so that although potatoes could be a good supply of aneurine, most of it is destroyed or lost in the cooking of this vegetable. The best way to eat potatoes is obviously to bake them in their jackets.

The practitioner will use it in all cases of deficiency and it must be remembered that although a daily requirement has been given, this is not a hard and fast rule as it is easily excreted and lost from the system, so that it is necessary to make sure that adequate amounts are properly assimilated. It is non-toxic and can be given in massive doses where these are required.

Riboflavine (Lactoflavine)

This is the name given to Vitamin "B"₂. Deficiency affects

the skin and can cause dermatitis, cracks at the corners of the mouth with inflammation of the lips. The cornea can be affected and become opaque with consequent loss of sight.

It occurs mostly in the products in which we find "B"$_1$ and to avoid the effects of too low a daily intake, foods rich in these vitamins must be taken regularly in the balanced diet. The average daily requirement is about $3\frac{1}{2}$ mg. but children require more, about 5 mg., as do expectant mothers.

Nicotinic Acid

This is called the P.P. or Pellagra Preventative Factor, and is widely used in the treatment of pellagra. A deficiency produces lassitude and weakness, with indigestion and in more chronic stages ulceration of the mouth, diarrhoea and a dermatitis of the exposed parts of the skin.

It is found always in close association with the other "B" group vitamins and a daily intake of approximately 50 mg. is necessary for health. It has the ability to dilate the arterioles and capillaries which must have a beneficial effect on the metabolism as far as the general distribution of nutrients is concerned, as well as the taking up of waste products for their eventual excretion. It is non-toxic in massive doses but if given in large doses on an empty stomach can cause erythema of the skin of the arms, face and across the back of the shoulders. Any patient should be warned of this possibility as the dose causing these symptoms (which are harmless) varies with different individuals and some do not experience them at all.

Pyrodoxin

This is Vitamin "B"$_6$ (adermin) and is needed by the body to maintain muscle tone. Deficiency of it is also a cause of anaemia. It is found in animal muscle and liver and also in fish, eggs, cereals and yeast. The daily requirement is around $2\frac{1}{2}$ mg. per day.

For the practitioner, it can be a useful aid in the treatment of Parkinson's Disease, paralysis agitans and muscular dystrophy and in all cases of lowered vitality.

Pantothenic Acid

This substance was originally thought to be responsible for affecting the pigment of the hair and that a deficiency would result in prematurely greying hair. However, this has now been somewhat discredited although it is still used in hair tonics for the promotion of healthy hair growth. In reality very little is known of the effects on human beings, but it is thought that an average daily diet should supply 6 mg. It may have something to do with sugar metabolism in humans but a great deal more research has to be done before anything concrete can be concluded as to the specific role of this vitamin in human nutrition.

Biotin

This has also been referred to as Vitamin "H" with pantothenic acid. It was at one time regarded as being a preserver of youth, but very little is known of the actual function of biotin or of the exact requirements. It too was associated with hair growth at one time. It is, however, certain that it is essential for many forms of plant and animal life and it can be concluded that it also has a vital use somewhere in the human metabolism.

Inositol and Choline

These are among the thermo stable "B" group of vitamins and do have rather different characteristics from the others. Again we can say very little about them in a factual way. Inositol is a kind of sugar like alcohol which occurs with linoleic acid and in this way may be useful in the treatment of some skin diseases. As research goes on continually into these complex products and their uses to man, the reader is urged to keep abreast of current findings by keeping up to date with every book which appears on this and allied subjects in the literature of biochemistry.

Para-amino Benzoic Acid

Yet another product of which very little is known. The

reader may remember that it received a great deal of publicity as a result of a Youth Elixir known as H3 "invented by a Professor Aslam from behind the Iron Curtain". H3 was reported to be procaine or novacaine (widely used by dentists for the relief of pain in tooth drilling). Procaine breaks down on ingestion to become the harmless para-aminobenzoic acid which has been known in England for many years. Its properties are relatively unknown. It too, no doubt, has a valuable part to play in human nutrition but little is known about it at the present time. Later reports stated that H3 combined this substance with assimilable potassium salts for the rejuvenation treatment and it is true that yeast (which contains a complexity of these "B" vitamin substances with protein) taken with assimilable potassium does have a good effect in maintaining health and vigour.

The results of our knowledge so far of these vitamins only goes to prove that we must ensure a good daily supply for although none of the extreme symptoms of deficiency may be present, there are on record many cases of "twilight" shortage which produce symptoms of varying degree in which the patient is never fully well. As these vitamins nearly always occur together in natural whole foods, it is fairly easy to prescribe a suitable diet when faced with any case of deficiency, however slight. In the more extreme cases they can always be prescribed in concentrated form as massive doses of yeast. Perhaps it is this that has led in recent years to yeast being hailed by one diet expert after another as a "wonder food"—but do not fall into the trap of thinking that any food is any more wonderful than any other. All foods play their important roles in a relative sense and all are equally useful in promoting life and preserving health and vitality, or of destroying it when taken to excess.

Vitamin "C"

This is probably the most widely known vitamin of all and one that the human body is totally unable to manufacture for itself or store in any quantity. Without it being present in the diet the disease known as scurvy manifests with all its unpleasant symptoms. So this vitamin is known as the anti-scorbutic vitamin. Chemically it has the name ascorbic acid. It controls the formation of intercellular substances like collagen in the capillary walls, dentine in teeth, cartilage and matrix in bone structure (osteoid tissue). It is a very valuable diuretic.

It is very necessary for the production of red corpuscles of the blood and transports hydrogen in the cells. Lack of this vitamin can produce a type of anaemia and the symptoms of scurvy are multiple haemorrhages which happen under the skin, in the joints and muscles. The classic example easily observed is bleeding of the gums with loosened teeth, the gums themselves becoming spongy.

In massive doses it can have an inhibiting effect on the growth of bacteria rather like penicillin. In other words it is bacteriostatic. But unlike penicillin with the use of ascorbic acid there is no harmful toxic result, no unpleasant side effects. It is widely used as a prophilactic against the common cold and against fevers, although more recent research seems to show that it has no effect on the virus of the common cold. A dose of 4 grammes at a time is required when used in this way. It is certainly useful in all infectious diseases and in diseases of the kidneys, etc. The average daily need is in the region of 50 mg. and should be rather more for children and old people.

A subnormal dose spread over many years may indeed be one of the predisposing factors in the various forms of arthritis, and this subnormal intake coupled with a shortage of physiological iron could perhaps be one of the predisposing factors to the prevalence of osteoid arthritis which is more common in older women than in men. The added drain on the organism during pregnancy could account for the prevalence in women.

The vitamin occurs in most fresh foods, including fresh meat, but as is wellknown, the main sources are blackcurrants, oranges, rose hips and other familiar fresh fruits.

The diet which includes a fair amount of fresh fruit and green vegetables will automatically provide the necessary amounts of ascorbic acid and only in deficiencies will it be necessary to resort to concentrated doses prepared in the laboratory or when it is being used as a bacteriostatic.

Vitamin "P"

This occurs in association with Vitamin "C" in all the citrus fruits. It is known as hesperidin (citrin). It can also be found in buck wheat and some other cereals such as RUTIN. It is essential in the human metabolic processes to prevent capillary fragility although in this respect some authorities have stated that ascorbic acid alone will do this.

There is still very little data on this vitamin but it does play an important part and especially in combination with Vitamin "C". Since it occurs so frequently with this latter, all the foods taken to provide a daily intake of ascorbic acid will also automatically give a good daily supply of citrin or rutin. Another source which should not be overlooked and which is an attractive addition to salads is paprika or Hungarian pepper.

The actual essential daily amount is not known but since it is non-toxic and in any case difficult to get under circumstances which would produce an overdose, no harm can be done by ensuring the patient takes large amounts of the fresh fruits, etc., in which it is found.

From this necessarily brief survey of vitamins and their place in human nutrition, we are able to work out the best diets for our individual requirements and we can use this knowledge to modify diets as and when required in relation to the condition being treated.

Although it may be argued that there is no need for any detailed knowledge of vitamins as these are bound to be provided in any good all-round diet, it is still a great advantage to be in a position to adjust the diet in relation to the condition being treated. With this specialized quantitative knowledge it is possible to regulate diet and treatment so that any additional synthetic micro nurients may be prescribed with qualitative and quantitative accuracy. In this way the optimum results are obtained in the shortest possible time.

CHAPTER 10

THE DUCTLESS GLANDS

Our main point in mentioning this system of glands is because the elements, vitamins and trace elements generally play a very large part in supplying the body with the raw material by which it can manufacture its own hormones which are the secretions of these glands.

There are two glandular systems in the human body. The one system has ducts which convey their secretions directly to the organs and the other is known as the ENDOCRINE or ductless system. These ductless glands, which are controlled by the pituitary gland (hence the name) secrete their hormones directly into the blood stream.

These hormones are vital secretions affecting the whole of our life processes and are intimately connected with growth and health. Many scientists have thought that by influencing hormone secretion in one way or another the life span and youth of the individual could be prolonged. The name of Voronoff and his sex gland grafts immediately springs to mind in this respect. Later the use of the male hormone testosterone became fashionable for those seeking renewed youth and many other substances with similar characteristics to testosterone have been marketed and used for the same purpose. Wasted and ageing muscles were said to be renewed with these substances but alas! after many years of use and hope, there does not seem to be much justification in the original wild claims. The undisputed facts still remain—it is only by maintaining the body in its totality in a healthful condition that health and prolonged activity can be maintained. All this brings us to a return to those great principles of Nature Cure first propounded by its pioneers. Certainly not one hormone, or glandular extract can be more rejuvenating than another and not one wonder food can claim to be the elixir that is better than all others. The health of our endocrine glands and indeed of our whole body depends on the totality of optimum measures taken for its continued health and well-being.

All these glands, like the rest of the human organism, depend for their efficient functioning on the correct daily intake of those vital micro nutrients with which we have dealt in the previous chapters. There is no other way to health and long life.

It is only in this general context that we now mention the various endocrine glands and some of the specific effects they have on our health. The failing of one will naturally affect the rest as they are interdependent on each other and all in turn are entirely dependent on a healthy blood supply properly equipped to carry full and adequate nutrition to every part of the body as well as being entirely efficient in carrying away the waste products and the residues left over from metabolism.

The Pituitary Gland

This is the governing factor of all the ductless glands. It has been called the conductor of the endocrine orchestra. It needs carbon, hydrogen, nitrogen, oxygen as well as sulphur, phosphorus and potassium.

The Pancreas

This gland in reality belongs to both glandular systems. It secretes insulin for which it too needs carbon, hydrogen, nitrogen, oxygen and sulphur. It regulates the sugar metabolism of the body.

The Gonads

These, vital to virility and reproduction, secrete mainly *Testosterone* and *Oestrin*. They also require carbon, hydrogen and oxygen. It is possible that they regulate deposits of fatty tissue in the male.

The Ovaries

The female counterpart of the Testis, they secrete the female hormones oestrin and androsterone which need carbon, hydrogen and oxygen for their formation.

Adrenal Medulla

This secretes adrenaline which can raise the blood pressure by having a constricting effect on the smaller arteries (arterioles). They are situated close to the kidneys.

Cortex

They secrete corticosterone and once again need carbon, nitrogen, hydrogen and oxygen in order to be able to do this.

Thyroid

This gland, which promotes and regulates growth, requires iodine in order to manufacture its secretion thyroxine, together with carbon, hydrogen, oxygen and nitrogen. This too has an effect on body weight and a sluggish thyroid can cause overweight while an overactive gland such as in conditions of hyperthyroidism can cause trembling symptoms, protruding eyes, etc.

Parathyroid

Little or nothing is known of this gland's secretions, but of course the same elements will be required for its efficient action.

The Thymus, Pineal Body and Spleen

Very little is known of these also at present other than that they too play a vital role in the metabolism. Disorders of the spleen can lead to constitutional blood diseases.

We are "as old as our glands" may or may not be true. We are as old as the sum total of all the tissues which go to make a human being. Without a constant and regular supply of correct nutrients, neither our glands nor any other tissues or structures of the body can maintain good health and efficient function. The shortage of any one of the vital nutrients which we have explained at length will lead in time to bad health and the interruption of the smooth running of any organism. Whether or not the ideal conditions of perfect environment coupled with perfect nutrition and perfect eliminative function will produce Eternal Youth is quite another question.

CHAPTER 11

TREATMENT BY FASTING

The Fast

Before going on to describe treatments involving specialized diets, it is logical first to describe treatments which are effective without food of any kind. In other words, treatments undertaken under conditions of fast.

Fasting is a form of curative treatment carried out in many Nature Cure establishments, but not so frequently attempted privately in the home. Naturally, in the Nature Cure resort the patient has the imposed discipline of the establishment to help him, and the task is therefore much easier than when a fast is undertaken in the freedom of one's own home. Also, the practitioner is able to see what day to day effects the fast has whereas he can never be absolutely sure if the patient is conscientiously carrying out the fast instructions when left to his own devices in his own house. A considerable amount of self-discipline is required of the patient or of anyone who wishes to undertake the rigours of a fast at home, as it is in cases of all restricted diets, but the value to the patient as an exercise in self-control, in addition to any physiological benefits which may accrue, is far greater than if he is supervised the whole time in an establishment where he cannot, if he wishes, depart from the regimen.

Many Naturopaths are inclined to exaggerate the importance of the fast and to prescribe a fast in all cases of illness. A study of what has been stated in previous chapters will prove the error of this. In all cases of serious deficiencies, a fast as such can only aggravate the condition, although it must also be admitted that in some cases there is need of a fast as well as the making good of deficiencies and in these cases it may be well to prescribe the most needed micro nutrients first before any kind of fast is undertaken.

A true fast consists of no food at all, and only water to be taken as required. The best effects of a fast can be obtained by observing this as far as solid food is concerned and allowing the patient only FRUIT JUICES. These can be given in diluted form. In this way the patient will receive some of the vital nutrients required while reaping the benefits of the fast.

Alterative Effect

The main effect of the fast is to have an alterative effect on the metabolism. This can also be effected with the aid of herbal remedies which are known in herbal medicine as alteratives and are indicated in all cases where an alterative effect is required and in which a fast would be harmful. An example of this is in emaciated cases which have undereaten so that a fast would be contra indicated.

The Initial Effects

The first effect of a complete fast is to make the patient feel much worse. This first stage, which usually lasts about three days, is the most critical. If the patient can survive these first few days with will-power and purpose intact, then the worst is over and good results will be evident afterwards. During these first days it is usual for the patient to experience headaches, fainting turns, lassitude and general debility. These symptoms come and go in cycles and it is the practitioner's duty to warn the patient in advance of what he may expect. This is the alterative effect getting under way. The first rush of elimination of toxins takes place and these circulating in the blood prior to being excreted under stimulation from the Vital Force produce the feeling of being worse than before.

The Enema

It is essential during the fast for the patient to take a gravity douche or enema every day in order to facilitate the elimination of waste products and toxins which are being churned up and

circulated. The first day should be commenced with an enema
of about 8 oz. of water at blood heat. The second day one
pint of water at the same temperature and the third, two pints.
This can be increased by one pint per day until a total of about
six pints has been reached and the patient should retain the
water for about half an hour, lying on the left side for the
reception of the water and then changing sides and lying on the
back for ten minutes each. The herbalist will prescribe herbal
infusions for this enema treatment during the fast and certainly
the addition of one or other of the indicated herbals in the
enema water as an infusion will be found of great benefit and
will add to the cleansing process.

Bath and Body Frictions

Although these will be dealt with fully under the subject of
Hydrotherapy, it is essential also for the patient to have a hot
bath followed by a cold immersion every day, and then good dry
frictions to the skin to stimulate elimination through this vital
organ.

Duration of the Fast

In general, for reasons already stated, a short fast or series
of short fasts are to be preferred to a long drawn out fast first
time which, under some circumstances, could seriously deplete
the patient and retard recovery. For instance, the strength of the
heart muscle could be undermined. Under no circumstances
take this risk and never prescribe a prolonged fast for a patient
undergoing this type of treatment at home. The practitioner
will be guided by the condition of the patient in determining
the actual length of even a short fast.

Restricted Diet

This may be found of most benefit to the patient at home
and especially the patient who must continue with some form
of routine activity during treatment. This would be prescribed
as follows:

On Rising—a glass of warm water with juice of a lemon.

Breakfast—2 slices of thin wholemeal toast lightly buttered, 2 apples or other fresh fruit in season.

Mid Morning—two glasses of water with an hour between each.

Midday—a silce of toast as before with a tomato and grated carrot or turnip (raw). Fresh fruit in season.

Mid Afternoon—two glasses of water as for mid-morning.

Tea—two thin slices of toast again with fresh fruit.

On Retiring—a glass of warm water with grape juice.

After the fourth day on this diet, gradually increase the balance of foods as required in each individual case, bearing in mind the weight, vitality and general condition of the patient.

General Uses of the Fast

Fasts are very necessary in the treatment of all disease where there is toxic accumulation and a general poisoning of the system, in all skin disorders, asthma, catarrhs and many digestive disturbances.

You will develop your own individual method and approach with practical experience and there is no doubt that it will soon be found possible to draw up competent diet sheets to suit any individual case. This is the main purpose of this book. It aims to inculcate an ability to deduct for yourself what is required in any given case. We do not give long lists of diseases with specific instructions as to which treatment may be the best. It is hoped that the intelligent use of the material found in this book will pave the way and lay the foundations from which the reader or practitioner will be able to evolve the best logical treatment for any and every condition presented in everyday life. Some patients will be found to be allergic to certain foods and there is no point, for instance, in insisting on orange juice or an orange cure for liver patients who cannot tolerate oranges (as so many naturopaths seem to do). Always gain the co-operation of the patient to be treated by taking him into your confidence and explaining things carefully as you go along. Nature Cure is not some hidden mystique but a sane and logical system of healing which can be straightforwardly explained to anyone.

That is why it is at the same time a good philosophy of general living which could and should be adopted by everyone.

Practitioners' Instructions

Always make these as clear and concise as possible commensurate with accuracy. Give detailed instructions of fast or restricted diet and set these out in a logical manner no matter how simple they may seem. (Some people have a gift for making the simple far too complicated.) Doing this will impress your patient and have the psychological effect of creating "faith" in you. This confidence which must be engendered is imperative if the treatment is to be successful and if the patient is to persevere through all the adverse symptoms which may attend the initial stages of a fast or restricted diet. Warn him in advance, do not let him think he is really getting permanently worse.

Food Temperatures

Always impress upon the patient the harm he can do by eating or drinking food which is too hot. There is even a theory and not without some foundation in fact, that hot food and drink acts as a carcinogenic irritant of the mouth and alimentary tract. This irritation causes loss of potassium which can have far reaching and adverse chronic effects on the health of the patient. Iced foods can have the same effect by cooling the system too rapidly, and it is known that these latter can so upset the intestinal tract as to cause acute inflammation of the appendix. It should also be pointed out that the intake during hot weather of such things as iced lollies and ice cream without an adequate protein diet can predispose towards such serious conditions as poliomyelitis. Always bear these things in mind when giving your patient instructions during treatment. Do not wonder what has happened to make the treatment ineffective if giving the proper introductory advice has been ignored.

Specialized Diets and Treatments

Many and varied specialized diets have been put forward

since Naturopathy was first used by the ancients as a true therapy. Of course, the intelligent practitioner will invent his own or modify the classical examples to his own individual requirements as and when modifications may be indicated in the individual case to be treated. One particular regimen that is worthy of our attention is known as the Schroth cure after the man who invented it and we will now deal with this important treatment.

The Schroth Cure—History

Johann Schroth was born in 1798 and brought up on his stepfather's farm at Lindweiss in Bohemia, or as it is now called, Czechoslovakia. From childhood his love of animals and his keen powers of observation led him to study the functioning of their bodies and to learn to understand their needs in health and sickness.

At the age of nineteen he was himself injured by a kick from a horse and discovered the use of the "wet pack" which he applied to his own badly damaged leg and healed it. He then further experimented on animals, treating their sufferings when wounded or injured or sick and effecting remarkably successful cures. From the use of the local wet pack for wounds, he developed the principle of the whole body pack, or Schroth Pack, which remains an essential feature of the SCHROTH TREATMENT. All the various methods used later with such success in healing the sick he first tried on himself, patiently and scientifically observing the effects.

Still observing animals in sickness, he experimented with FASTING, i.e. abstaining entirely from food during sickness in order to eliminate poisons from the body. Further acute observation led him to discover that THIRSTING—going without drink for long periods—was an even more effective treatment in curing chronic illness than fasting.

Illness he saw as a condition of stress and strain for the ailing body, taxing the body's physical endurance in much the same way as physical exercise. He had observed that animals doing hard physical work, e.g. horses ploughing, when given dry food with little to drink had far more endurance than when allowed to drink freely, when they perspired more and got tired sooner.

He applied this principle for developing the body's stamina in the struggle to overcome disease, and he found that the more the patient thirsted, the more rapidly the acids and toxins accumulated in the diseased body were loosened and expelled from the system, with a consequent return to health and vigour.

The literally acid test was in the urine of the patient which under his treatment revealed the enormous quantities of uric acid waste products which were being eliminated. One doctor who recently interested himself in this treatment, on being shown the urine specimens of patients, was absolutely amazed and remarked that in forty years of practice as a medical man he had never seen urine like it! He afterwards confessed that he was ashamed of his profession for closing its eyes to the results of this remarkable treatment.

Some liquid, however, is essential because the body becomes dehydrated very rapidly, and it was only after much experimenting with drinks of various kinds that Schroth finally decided on a light white wine as the ideal medium, partly because no other drink was found to be so successful in stirring up and eliminating the impurities which caused disease.

Schroth maintained that the primary cause of disease is not the bacteria and virus which are present in the symptoms manifested, but the accumulated impurities in the body caused by civilized man's eating habits. In this belief Johann Schroth was in harmony with all other pioneers of Naturopathy. He was and is unique.

His village of Lindweiss, or Dolni-Lipova as it is now re-named, lies tucked away among the Altvater mountains, as inaccessible and remote a place as can be imagined, reached only by a long and tedious train journey. Yet before the war more than 3,000 patients a year flocked to it to be treated. They were boarded out in the villagers' homes and other hostels, and the whole village life was regulated by the rhythm of the "Cure". Monday—Dry Day; Tuesday—Small Drink Day; Wednesday—

Dry Day; Thursday—Big Drink Day; Friday—Small Drink Day and during the week-end, Saturday—Small Drink Day; Sunday—Big Drink Day.

Not only the chronic sick from all over Europe and beyond, but also their relatives gladly made the long journey to this little "Mecca of the Uncured", some to seek the return of health and others to enjoy a holiday in the unique atmosphere of this quaint Bohemian village which was presided over by the benign genius of one of the greatest natural healers who has ever lived—Johann Schroth.

When Johann died, his son Emanuel, who ranks almost as highly as his father, followed on and did much to further develop and establish the "Cure". During a lifetime his father had been persecuted as a "quack" and even threatened with imprisonment, but in Emanuel's day some of the more far-sighted medical men began to take notice and from this time forward the reputation of the treatment was established beyond doubt.

At the end of World War II, Schroth's village lay in ruins, sacked by the Russians on their way into Germany, but the doctors who had been in charge since the last of the Schroth brothers had passed on, had fled and spread their knowledge with them. Today Schroth Centres exist in Obervellach in Austria and the Oberstaufen in Germany, and the treatment is practised in several hospitals in that country. In Czechoslovakia the desecration of the village has been amply atoned for by the inclusion of the Schroth treatment in their National Health Service—an example all would do well to follow. It is also in Czechoslovakia that (while many of the spas in countries like England are faded relics of Victorian opulence) they continue to flourish and offer treatment by radioactive mud packs and many other natural means. Many of the famous Czechoslovakian spas are too well-known to require mention here and the work they do in the cause of health is known far beyond the boundaries of that little country. The sick and desperately ill from many outside countries, particularly from the Federal Republic of Western Germany, still flock to these spas for treatments that have stood the test of time and will outlast the vogue of all the wonder drugs.

It may be possible to exploit the people for some of the time by offering wonder drugs and welfare state schemes based on big vested interests, but the laws of preservation and survival will certainly insist that sooner or later more notice must be taken of these natural treatments than is currently being done in the opulent countries of the Western World where every new "gimmick" can bring a fortune for its inventor.

CHAPTER 12

THE SCHROTH CURE

The Importance of Diet

Those who will derive most benefit from the Schroth treatment are those suffering from the rheumatic and arthritic complaints—fibrositis, sciatica, lumbago, etc., and those leading sedentary occupations where little or no exercise and overeating is coupled with the stresses and strains of modern living—in short the executive office types. Dropsical conditions with excess body fluids will also benefit. In carrying out this treatment it is essential to understand that once the toxins have been eliminated and the metabolism restored to normal, a diet rich in foods which will produce an alkaline reaction in the body is to be adhered to. This is also true of the diet used in preparation for the Schroth treatment itself.

The most important foods which do produce an alkaline reaction in the body are the fresh *acid fruits* and second to these are fresh non-starchy green and root vegetables. In the fruit category we are not, of course, referring to dried oily fruits such as dates, figs, walnuts and other nut kernels, nor do we mean bananas. In the vegetable group we omit parsnips which are starchy and potatoes which have about 15 per cent starch. Carrots and white turnips are the best root vegetables for our purpose, and fruits as they may be in season are apples, pears, peaches, apricots, oranges, grapefruit and lemons (the latter are particularly good). If the vegetables are to be taken cooked, they should be conservatively cooked. On no account should salt ever be used in the preparation of any special diet. To cook the vegetables, have a minimum quantity of water brought to the boil and then place the washed, prepared vegetables in the boiling water and simmer just long enough to soften them. They are then ready to eat and will taste a great deal better than those prepared in the more orthodox way.

The preparation diet should consist of a preponderance of the above-mentioned foods, and protein foods at this stage should be kept at a minimum. They are of course the meats, fish, mushrooms, yeasts, nuts, eggs, cheese, etc.

Make sure the patient has WHOLE FOODS if possible, fresh from their source of growth, and again if at all possible those grown on naturally composted soil or fed on foods from such soil in the case of animal meat.

Foods to Avoid

White sugar and white flour are a scourge to our civilization. They and their products are to be avoided at all costs. Never on any account allow the patient to have anything of this nature as in so doing the work of months can be ruined in a few weeks. Under this heading are, of course, the jams, conserves, honey (where the bees are fed on white sugar), sweets, white bread, cake, pastry and all synthetic soft drinks.

Drinks

The instructions given here in connection with the Schroth Cure are equally suitable as preparative measures for any other specialized treatment such as the mono diet, etc., and indeed the doctrine of WHOLE FRESH FOODS is one of the foundation stones of Naturopathic Philosophy in Practice. All patients should be carefully told of the advantages to their health in the long term if these simple rules are followed. It is useless being cured of one condition if immediately afterwards there is to be a return to the old harmful ways of living, including eating.

Tea, coffee and alcoholic drinks are the social evils of our time. We all know the business executive who will tell you that he cannot avoid numberless cups of tea and many whiskies during a day in order to better entertain his business associates. This also applies to the habit of smoking. If these people could only be persuaded that less earnings would be preferable and would not mean less of the really good things of life, for they would need a lot less by way of expenses and earnings if they cut out their weekly bills for these social "gimmicks"! A cup of freshly made weak tea or a pleasant cup of coffee taken when really thirsty is harmless as is a pleasant glass of light grape wine, but to take these things for any reason other than genuine thirst or need is stupid and only works the organism for nothing, apart from the toxic effects they produce which cannot be overcome by any but the hardest manual workers.

Authorities vary in their pronouncements as to the amount of liquid required by an individual in any one day, and amounts ranging from one to five pints have been put forward. This must naturally depend to a large extent on the nature of the work done and the climate in which one lives. In this preparative diet between 1 and 1½ pints is quite enough.

With these basic ideas in mind, we now give the average daily intake of food which should be continued for a week or even two weeks according to the state of health of the patient before the actual Schroth treatment is embarked on.

Given this preparative diet guide, the intelligent practitioner will be able to work out several alternatives and the following is only given as a general guidance. With a special case in hand, specialized adaptations can be worked out, but always make sure that the patient is fully aware of what is involved and that he understands completely all the instructions given and the reasons for giving them.

The Diet Chart (General)

ON RISING—a teaspoonful of pure honey (preferably from wild bees and certainly not from those fed on white sugar. It is thought that foreign honey may be better than English in this respect as in most cases English bees are fed on white sugar through the winter months). Take this in a glass of warm water, with a tablespoonful of lemon juice. Pure blackcurrant juice would make a good alternative to the lemon juice.

BREAKFAST—fresh chopped apples with soaked raisins to

which has been added a teaspoonful of wheat germ (this can be obtained under the trade names of Bemax or Froment).

or

Soaked dried prunes and grated apple with wheat germ. To prepare the raisins, pour boiling water over enough for the breakfast the night before and leave overnight. Use the liquor with the breakfast dish. Prunes should be soaked overnight in the same way.

MID-MORNING—a cup of freshly made weak tea (without sugar) or glass of fresh fruit juice.

LUNCHEON—this should be a salad meal consisting of fresh leafy vegetables in season such as lettuce, endive, fresh chopped young cabbage, watercress, etc., with two root vegetables freshly grated, such as carrot, turnip and celery. Chopped chives, onion or garlic may be used in place of condiments. A baked jacket potato may be taken with this meal and fresh lean meat (cold) or grated cheese or hard boiled eggs.

MID-AFTERNOON—a glass of fresh fruit juice or cup of freshly made weak tea, unsweetened.

EVENING MEAL—this may be a cooked meal consisting of roast or stewed meat, steamed fish or poached eggs with jacket potato and one fresh green leafy vegetable with two root vegetables in season, cooked as described in a conservative manner. The vegetable water, if any is left, should be used in conjunction with the meal as a gravy.

N.B. The lunch and evening meals may be interchanged for convenience, and in both cases the sweet should consist of fresh raw fruit in season or yoghourt. In the case of overweight patients, Marmite or Yeastrel may be used with the vegetable water to make the gravy, for the cooked meal.

When using meat, always remember to boil this for two minutes and then throw the water away before cooking it for use or roasting it. In this way the water soluble toxic substances will be removed and this is most important in the case of rheumatic sufferers.

As a change, the cooked meal can also include a really good vegetable and meat stock soup, but make it fresh and do not keep it for any length of time and certainly not for future use. In cases of lowered vitality and where there are no other contra-indications, a little fresh cream may be taken with the fresh fruit dessert. In addition to the condiments mentioned, parsley will be found of great value in cases of urinary tract disturbances.

Now to the basis of the SCHROTH CURE ITSELF.

A Schroth Dry Day

It must again be emphasized that perseverence is essential if any good is to come of a sound naturopathic regimen. Emanuel Schroth always held the following motto before his patients. It is well worth quoting here—

> "Without battle—no victory,
> Without self-denial—no satisfaction,
> Without cleansing—no healing."

When the patient has been on the preparation diet for one to three weeks as thought necessary, a first attempt at a dry day may be made as a trial without the use of the WET PACK (which is an essential part of the Schroth Cure and on which we shall enlarge later).

ON RISING—rinse the mouth with apple juice (but drink nothing).

BREAKFAST—dry toast, NO BUTTER—NOTHING ELSE.

LUNCH—dry toast or stale rolls—NOTHING ELSE.

EVENING—one half pint of pure apple juice or dry white French wine.

The following morning the preparation diet can be continued as before. This dry day is just another part of the preparation of the patient for the complete SCHROTH CURE.

Incidentally, in many cases which may not require the full SCHROTH TREATMENT a DRY DAY at intervals will help considerably with any form of Naturopathic Treatment, and has been found to precipitate a healing crisis. These dry days carefully graduated can often assist in bringing about a cure of the less serious cases while the patient is not incapacitated in any way and able to continue as nearly a normal daily life as possible.

The dry day can be taken say once weekly, spread over a long period where necessary. It is especially good in cases of sluggish lymphatics where fluid accumulates in the body and the patient is liable to swelling of joints at frequent intervals.

The Strict Treatment

This is the most drastic and effective known method for the elimination of uric acid from the body. It is for this reason it achieves such striking results in all the rheumatic and arthritic cases. The alternating "dry" and "drink" days draw the acids out of the tissues back into the blood stream whence they can be eliminated naturally via the kidneys (by flushing with wine) and through the skin (with the aid of WET PACKS). The quantities of uric acid deposits in the urine during a Schroth course need to be seen to be believed. It can be a long process getting rid of these accumulated deposits from the system and some patients will need to persevere through perhaps two full Schroth Treatments or even more, with intervals on a less restrictive diet between. In any case the patient will be encouraged to persevere as considerable relief will be obtained quite early in the treatment, and certainly the inflammations with their attendant pain will subside.

The True Wet Pack Treatment

This pack should be applied every night during the Schroth Treatment, but it is rightfully a part of Hydrotherapy and is included under that section of the book, where it is fully explained. To save space and avoid repetition, it is not given here. This section of the book dealing as it does with details of human nutrition leaves enough for the reader to absorb without changing subjects in mid-stream as it were. It will be quite a simple matter to co-ordinate the WET PACK with the dietetic part of this treatment when the chapter on Hydrotherapy has also been fully studied. Meanwhile, it is best to concentrate on the dietetics of the Schroth Treatment. But please remember that this treatment is in no way complete without the application of the WET PACK every night of the Cure.

Bearing this in mind, we continue now with full details of the day-to-day diet of the Schroth Treatment which in its complete cycle lasts for one week. As stated before, several cycles can be used at intervals in difficult and obstinate cases, and although many cases will respond completely after only one cycle, there are many chronic sufferers who will only obtain the maximum benefit from this treatment by undergoing more than one cycle, but always with a suitable interval on a restricted diet in between.

Schroth Strict Regimen

Monday	*Tuesday*	*Wed-nesday*	*Thursday*	*Friday*	*Satur-day*	*Sunday*
	SMALL		BIG		SMALL	BIG
DRY	DRINK	DRY	DRINK	DRY	DRINK	DRINK
DAY	DAY	DAY	DAY	DAY	DAY	DAY
Breakfast 2 large slices dry toast	*Breakfast* As Monday	*throughout*	*Breakfast* As Monday	*throughout*	*throughout*	*throughout*
Midday Dry stale rolls as required all day	*Midday* 1 plate porridge	*As Monday*	*Midday* Baked potato with boiled onions, 3 or 4 according to size; 7 dry prunes	*As Monday*	*As Tuesday*	*As Thursday*

Monday	Tuesday	Wed-nesday	Thursday	Friday	Satur-day	Sunday
	SMALL		BIG		SMALL	BIG
DRY	DRINK	DRY	DRINK	DRY	DRINK	DRINK
DAY	DAY	DAY	DAY	DAY	DAY	DAY
3 p.m.	*3 p.m.*		*3 p.m.*			
ditto	Half bottle dry white wine to last until bedtime		Up to 1 full bottle dry white wine to last until bedtime			
Evening ditto	*Evening* ditto		*Evening* ditto			
Bedtime Full body WET PACK	*Bedtime* As Monday	As Monday throughout	*Bedtime* The pack may be missed one day weekly on a big drink day	As Monday throughout	As Tuesday throughout	As Thursday throughout

CHAPTER 13

MONO DIETS

For many years it has been known that periods on an exclusive food with absolutely nothing else with the exception of liquids will produce very beneficial results in cases of chronic disease conditions, and it is true that many people owe their lives and restored health to perseverence through long periods on a mono diet of one kind or another. A mono diet can become very tedious and monotonous but the results obtained are more than enough to offset any mental depression which may be a psychological side effect or would be in the absence of encouraging symptoms which often manifest themselves in a very short time.

One of the reasons for the success of the mono diet is that the stomach has only one kind of food on which to work and which only takes a given time to digest, after which the bodily energies are conserved, having obtained the maximum nutrition from the food ingested. Elimination is also encouraged to a degree not possible with more varied diets, however "balanced" they are. Thus it can be seen that for the emaciated patient who is undernourished in the true sense of the world, a period on a suitable mono diet would be much more desirable than a fast, however short it may be.

The practitioner must at all times be guided by the condition of the patient and by his own tests and observations before deciding which treatment is to be the best for the case with which he is concerned. All the treatments outlined here are good, but not necessarily good for every case. The skill and competence of a good practitioner is always required to make the decision on correct treatment. If this were not so, the patient could pick up the nearest book advocating Naturopathy and commence at

once on any fad or fancy put forward with the hope of successful cure. We all know that this can never be, and Naturopathy
is often brought into disrepute by readers of popular magazines
doing just this. The result is that the magazines which are so
keen on converting members of the public to the Naturopathic
system of healing often, in fact, fail miserably and send their
readers straight back to allopathic treatments because it is all
made to sound so very simple and quickly effective when this is
very often not the case.

These treatments, although they are simple in themselves, do
need the experience of the properly trained practitioner to
supervise and prescribe the correct kind of treatment for the
particular case. If the patient is intent on self-treatment, then a
study of the sound basic principles of Naturopathic Practice
such as are given in the present book are required so that the
most suitable individual treatment can be worked out and
followed conscientiously by the ordinary intelligent person. It is
useless to write a list of disease syndromes and then to say that a
fast followed by a balanced diet will CURE EVERYTHING. It is
also useless to think that a mono diet, however skilfully applied,
will be successful in the cure of every disease, and the same is
true of every other therapy, no matter under which school of
medicine it is practised. Natural treatments will always be
effective when used with skill and intelligence by a competent
practitioner or anyone who studies the subject fully and carefully
and realizes the obvious limitations in each therapy and that
different therapies have different applications. Allopathic drug
therapy can never be successful in any true sense of the word
"cure" for this very reason—it never attempts to put the whole
of the body in a state of harmonious health but specializes in
the suppression of the presently manifesting symptoms of which
the patient for the time being complains. Not to worry if these
symptoms having been suppressed, the patient is then afflicted
with another set of symptoms resulting from the side effects
of the treatment which "cured" the first set.

When studying the different therapies outlined in this book

it is well to bear in mind these facts and never to place over-importance on one set of treatments as distinct from others. All have their correct uses under given conditions and the secret is in the co-ordination of compatible treatments to secure a complete eradication of the causes of the disease at the earliest possible moment without in any way attempting to suppress the symptoms which in any event will merely have the effect of laying down the preconditions of more chronic disease to follow. The primary object of Naturopathy is not only to cure but to educate the patient thereafter to live in accordance with principles which will ensure that he will remain active, alert and in the best possible health during a life which is as long and full as possible.

The Grape Cure

This is universally known and widely used in the treatment of chronic disease. It is popular all over Europe and in the United States of America. There are many institutions which exist only to carry out the grape cure. It is a wonderful remedy for all the rheumatic complaints by virtue of its high content of acids and organic mineral matter. It also supplies valuable micro nutrients to the nervous system so often fatigued and depicted as a result of the rheumatic symptoms and effects.

In prescribing the Grape Cure, it is essential to place the patient on a preparation diet first, and for this the reader can refer back to that given under the instructions for the Schroth Cure. It is sound preparation diet for any mono cure. The practitioner using this as a foundation can always modify it in detail to include a predominance of the nutrients required for the particular case or select foods having therapeutic properties which are required.

Assuming then that the patient has been properly prepared and the necessary enemas have been given during a preliminary three or four day fast following the preparation diet in the case of overweight patients, then immediately after the fast commence with the first day of $1\frac{1}{2}$ lb. of fresh grapes. This amount is increased by $\frac{3}{4}$ to 1 lb. daily according to the desire or the need on the part of the patient to eat. No other food or drink is permitted. The increase will be continued each day until the patient is taking some 12 lb. of grapes. The maximum quality should be continued for twelve to fourteen days, during which time the patient will also undergo various hydrotherapy or osteopathy treatments as may be indicated—local packs, frictions and compresses, etc., with good general massage and soft tissue manipulation, etc. These special water and manipulative treatments are described in later chapters.

Mono diets in respect of other fruits can also be carried out. The fruit chosen is the one having the properties, both therapeutic and nutrient, which will be most suited to the cases being treated.

THE ORANGE DIET—very useful in all cases of auto intoxication.

THE APPLE—another mono diet for the rheumatic sufferers, when apples are in season. It is rich in phosphorus for the nerves, and malic acid which will dissolve deposits of lime in the joints. It is also a powerful antiseptic in the body like LEMON.

THE PEAR—another rich source of phosphorus, iron and sodium salts.

THE STRAWBERRY—although having a limited season in this country, it is valuable as a mono diet, especially in the acute and painful type of rheumatism. It contains natural salicin (not the derivative of coal tar as are aspirin tablets) as well as iron and silicon with calcium.

THE BILBERRY—this is a useful blood purifier and is thus a valuable alterative. It is a good treatment for eczemas and other skin diseases. Blackcurrants, redcurrants and raspberries are also good for skin affections and are rich in magnesia, lime and iron.

Vegetable Mono Diets

Certain vegetables are also ideal when used as mono diets and celery is an example of this in the treatment of rheumatic complaints of long standing and where these occur in middle age and where there is premature ageing. Celery is also extremely valuable for sexual deficiency and impotence in the male. The hearts should be cleaned and chopped and eaten fresh and raw When a vegetable diet such as this is undertaken, it is quite permissible to prescribe a suitable fruit juice for liquid intake or where this is not advisable, fresh water. If fruit juice is prescribed, it should be emphasized that an interval of about an hour should elapse between eating the vegetable and taking the fruit juice.

The Acids of Fresh Fruits

The following are the principal acids of the more common fruits which will be of help in deciding which may be the best for the required mono diet.

MALIC ACID—it is useful as a stimulant of gastric secretions. It also assists in the elimination of accumulated toxins and is of great value in chronic diseases. It is found in the following fruits: apples, plums, pears, tomatoes, cherries, cranberries, strawberries, gooseberries and grapes.

CITRIC ACID—useful for liver complaints, rheumatic disorders, neuritis, feverish conditions, etc. It is present in all the citrus fruits—lemons, oranges, grapefruit and pomegranates. For other reasons the orange may be contra indicated in liver conditions while grapefruit and its juice are wonderful in cases of inflammation of the gall bladder and gall stones.

OXALIC ACID—the vegetables rich in this acid are usually of help in restoring vitality and in anaemic conditions. They are: spinach, rhubarb, sorrel, cocoa, tea, pepper, etc.

RENSOIC ACID—this is an acid which must never be prescribed in excess. It is present in plums, prunes and cranberries. It prevents swift putrefaction.

TARTARIC ACID—another acid useful in the rheumatic complaints and present in grapes.

More Fruits and Vegetables and Their Uses

In order to make this list as complete as possible, the more well-known fruits and vegetables are listed below with indications of their value and hints for use. They can be incorporated not only into the specialized mono diets with which we are dealing, but the information here given will be found invaluable in using these foods by taking advantage of their special indications and specific effects in certain diseases in more general diets. In this way more generalized diets for long continued use can be worked out and these used in conjunction with herbal or homeopathic remedies as well as the external treatments—hydrotherapy and physiotherapy—mentioned earlier for a restoration of health in the shortest possible time. Never be unilateral in the uses of or in the application of natural therapeutics.

GRAPEFRUIT—very useful in cases of liver disorders of all kinds. It is of benefit in feverish conditions and has a mild, natural laxative action.

PEACHES—these should be included in all diets where there is disorder of the kidneys or where there is urinary tract infection. Copious draughts of the juice prove a good means of flushing and cleansing the urinary tract. Also useful in cases of dysentery.

PINEAPPLE—this is a singularly useful fruit in the hands of a good naturopath. It is said that the juice of the pineapple will dissolve the membrane of diphtheria and it is certainly a wonderful remedy for all inflammatory conditions of the throat and of the alimentary tract generally. For this reason it is extremely useful in all digestive disorders.

TOMATOES—although in reality a vegetable by classification, these can be included with the fruits. Useful in kidney malfunction. There is only one drawback to the use of these and that is the fact that most tomatoes are so far from being a natural product these days that it is sometimes wise to avoid them. They are in the main artificially produced and forced for early markets, etc., grown mainly under glass in the country, which does form an insulator for much cosmic radiation. It is because of this that many people prefer them for the table as their skins are so much softer than the more naturally grown outdoor variety, but this is not a recommendation of their therapeutic value.

CARROTS—rich in the precursor of Vitamin "A", Carrotene, they are also rich in iron and other minerals which make them useful in the treatment of ulcerated conditions and again in kidney disease. For ulcers that refuse to heal, try a poultice of raw carrots changed daily.

LETTUCE—also rich in iron and has a sedative effect. Its use in the diet when properly masticated will help in nervous afflictions as well as kidney complaints.

SPINACH—one of the best vegetable sources of iron. It is a good laxative and a valuable addition to the diet of the anaemic and liverish.

ONIONS—with onions we may also include garlic, which promotes the elimination of uric acid and so is good for rheumatic sufferers. Garlic was used many centuries B.C. as a treatment for rheumatic affections by nations in the Near and Middle East. It is also of great value in soothing inflammations of all the membranous linings of the body and in this way is invaluable in the treatment of bronchitis. To make a really effective remedy for bronchitis and as a soothing alleviation of all types of cough, cover a saucer of chopped onion with honey and leave overnight suitably covered. Pour off the liquor the next morning and take a teaspoonful every two or three hours.

BEET TOPS—these boiled are a useful remedy for bladder disorders and for gravel or stones. Bruise a pound of the leaves and pour on them $1\frac{1}{2}$ pints of boiling water. Simmer slowly until there is a pint of decoction left. Allow to cool and strain when cold. Take a wineglass every hour or more often throughout the day. Make a fresh supply every two days. They can also be included as a vegetable in the diets of these sufferers.

POTATOES—rich in the "B" group of vitamins and in sodium and potassium salts. They assist in the elimination of uric acid from the system and are another good remedy for rheumatism. They can be used very well with modifications of the Schroth Cure by substituting the baked jacket potato for dry toast. Make sure the potatoes are really well baked for this purpose.

The Milk Diet

The exclusive milk diet is given here with many mixed feelings. Very unfortunately, milk today is only very rarely obtainable in its fresh natural state. It is far more frequently anything but whole fresh milk, being pasteurised after being obtained from herds of cows developed by various artificial means to give the maximum quantity yield. Some of these measures include the use of massive doses of various antibiotics which are all too frequently measurable in the milk. Milk too is a mucin forming food and can increase the chronicity of catarrhal conditions. Since, however, it does form a part of accepted naturopathic practice, we include it here under the mono diets since, if fresh whole milk can be obtained directly from properly fed herds of good sound stock, then it may undoubtedly be of great value in the treatment of a whole range of chronic disease conditions. If the fresh whole unpasteurised milk cannot be obtained, it is better to use one of the fruit mono diets in its place.

Before discussing milk as a mono diet, we may mention here the value of BUTTERMILK with a potato diet in the treatment of rheumatic and arthritic conditions. Do not despair with a case of chronic rheumatism or arthritis until this TWO FOOD diet has been well and truly tested. It nearly always produces astounding results.

Milk taken fresh from the animal is a food at nearly human vibration. It will imbue the cells with renewed vitality without any great efforts on the part of the metabolism in digestion. It has for many years been used with wonderful results in Russia and Germany and the Balkan countries. In addition to being easily digested, it is rich in most nutrients—proteins, fats, elements, salts, vitamins and enzymes. It can be used without fear of the patient becoming undernourished in any way. It is an almost complete food so that while enjoying the benefits of complete nutrition, the patient is also having the full physiological advantage of a mono diet. Naturally, it is best undertaken when milk is at its best. This is in the spring or at least during the summer season when the cows are enjoying the free range of open pastures.

The optimum amount of milk for the daily intake is in the region of six quarts. This should be built up after the patient has been on the preparation diet for two or three weeks. A short fast may also be an advantage after the preliminary diet. The fast undertaken should not be of long duration—of about four or five days at most, during which time the full enema or gravity douche treatment should be given.

The first day of the All-Milk Diet should consist of a pint sipped very slowly (and chewed in the mouth before swallowing) at midday. Another pint should be taken in the same way at about 6 p.m. and nothing else for the whole day. The next day double this amount of milk is taken at three different meals. Gradually increase this on succeeding days until a maximum of six quarts is being consumed daily. This should then be continued as a staple diet for perhaps two or three weeks according to the case and how it responds.

The diet is broken by including half the amount of milk on the first day of departure from the All-Milk intake and an amount of approximately 1 lb. of freshly grated carrots or celery —again prescribed according to the indications of the particular case—after two or three more days, additional fresh foods can be introduced until a balanced all-round diet is achieved which can then be continued indefinitely.

During the period of the All-Milk Diet, the necessary auxiliary treatments such as hydrotherapy, physiotherapy, etc., should be carried out to stimulate circulation, breathing, etc., which will speed up the metabolism with a consequent acceleration of the elimination of poisons and waste products from the system.

For lowered vitality and poor muscle tone, the milk diet is unrivalled. It has been known to cure cases of constipation of many years standing. This happens when the effects of the scorifying products usually taken by the uninformed layman have been removed. Make sure the patient never again resorts to the use of dangerous bowel irritants. These irritants only work in ever increasing doses, destroying the muscle tone of the bowel in such a way that in the end they become completely ineffective, however large the dose taken. This is no cure for constipation and can be most certainly the cause of auto-intoxication as very often the patient, thinking that the irritant laxative is doing its job, is not aware that it is merely liquifying a small content of the intestine while large amounts of dried and hardened waste products are left over very long periods attached to the bowel membrane, being partially re-absorbed into the system and causing poisoning in this way.

The success of true health depends on proper assimilation of all the nutrients required by the body for its work and self-repair in addition to successful and complete elimination of ALL waste products and toxins which will otherwise accumulate in the system and slow down metabolism causing chronic disease of every conceivable kind.

Yogurt, Sour Milk and Buttermilk

This chapter on milk as a food would not be complete without some mention of Yogurt. Many years ago it was thought that Yogurt was the secret of prolonged youth and an aid to a very long active life, in addition to being a detoxicant of the system. The reasons given for this belief were that people whose diet contained large quantities of yogurt were very strong, very fit and lived to ripe old ages, and in fact, regions where this food was supposed to have been consumed as a main part of the diet to have large populations of virile old people. These are the peasant populations of the Balkan countries and Russia. It was also stated that Yogurt had the properties necessary for the destruction of the germs and bacteria which attacked mankind, bringing about plagues and epidemics of all kinds. It is recorded that the great Russian scientist Metchnikof, lecturing to students on these matters one day, in full view of his class, is reputed to have swallowed a vial of active cholera germs as proof of the protection he had obtained by eating large amounts of yogurt. At all events, it is true that Metchnikof did not catch cholera, but he was dead at the age of 60 which does not say much for the longevity producing powers of this food. Later investigators also found that the peasants of these countries did not eat yogurt so much as just ordinary soured milk. Milk soured in a special way—not allowed to turn sour in a cupboard but soured in the sunlight. Their milk was not, of course, pasteurised and their sour milk or yogurt was always prepared from fresh, whole milk. These ideas on the attributes of such milk products apart, it is beyond doubt that they do have a very valuable part to play in dietetics and they do contain properties of immense therapeutic value.

Buttermilk, sour milk and yogurt are rich in lactic acid which is also produced by the body from the fermentation of sugars by certain enzymes. This acid is very valuable in the colon as it prevents harmful putrefaction of waste products.

These milk products are also valuable to the vegetarian as sources of protein. Yogurt, particularly that made from goat's milk as obtained in Greece, Turkey and the Balkan countries, is always a very useful item in any sound diet.

CHAPTER 14

THE ALL-MEAT DIET

An all-meat or all-fish diet has been used mostly in the treatment of wasting disease. It was originated by a Dr. Salisbury about the middle of the nineteenth century. It can be very valuable for depleted vitality and in all cases of faulty assimilation. It is particularly helpful in cases involving the aged. It is a very easily digested food which is readily available for the body's needs and as was explained in earlier chapters on food classification, it contains those first class proteins which the body can so easily use to make and build so many of the vital substances required for day-to-day existence as well as to combat disease.

In using meat for an exclusive diet, it should always be fresh and should be cooked in the minimum amount of water. For therapeutic purposes, it should never be roasted or cooked in any other way. Here we must repeat the instruction for the preparation of meat given earlier. IT MUST ALWAYS BE BOILED FOR TWO MINUTES AND THE WATER THROWN AWAY BEFORE BEING PREPARED FOR FOOD. It is only by doing this that the harmful toxinous effects of meat eating can be avoided. No matter whether you are well or ill, this pre-boiling should always be carried out before meat is ever used for human consumption.

It is logical that this type of diet cannot in the strict sense of the word be termed "mono" as the patient will always require a liquid intake in addition to the meat. This can be taken as water at blood temperature or fruit juice at the same temperature. Fruit juice is by far the more satisfactory as it does for all practical purposes supply the complement of meat in human nutrition. The knowledge gained in the preceding chapter regarding the relative values and therapeutic uses of fruit juices will be used here when arriving at a choice of fruit for this purpose.

The fat and gristle should be removed from the meat for the purpose of this diet and boiling water poured over it, when it is simmered until tender enough to eat. (This is AFTER the previous boiling when the water is thrown away.) Do not use salt or any other substance in the cooking and do not cook in aluminium or stainless steel utensils. Enamelled pans are best.

As in all other exclusive diets, the patient must be prepared for it in a proper manner with a preparatory diet followed where indicated by a short fast and the gravity douche treatment.

When the patient is ready, the meat, minced so as to be even more readily digested, is given on the first day following the preparation. A quarter of a pound of meat forms the first meal which is at midday. The meat is thoroughly mixed with the saliva before swallowing and is eaten as slowly as possible. The meat does not in reality digest in the mouth and the slow mastication is here recommended in order that the stomach shall receive it as slowly as possible.

About an hour after or an hour before this midday meal, a glass of fruit juice is taken and again at intervals between the meals of meat.

The next meal is identical to the first. The same amount of meat taken at about 6 p.m. This will complete the first day with the fruit juice or warm water as described.

The second day the meals are increased from two to three by introducing a morning meal. Otherwise the regimen is the same.

The third day the amount of meat at each meal is increased to a total of a pound and a quarter for the day. From then on for the next two or three weeks, as long as the all-meat diet is continued, a total of two pounds by weight pre-cooked of the meat may be taken each day.

When the time comes for the introduction of a more complete and balanced diet, vegetables can be introduced daily and later a little wholemeal bread.

An all-meat diet is important in the case of diabetes, stomach complaints, constipation, Bright's Disease and many others. It can also be modified to a two-part diet by including an appropriate vegetable such as carrot or celery.

Modifications

For those patients who are obese and cannot take carbohydrate even in small quantities without gaining weight, a meat and fat diet is of great importance. The fat will provide the calories for this type of patient without increasing weight. It should, however, be borne in mind that a variety of fats should be included in this type of diet and not purely animal fat. Oils such as sunflower seed oil, corn oil and other vegetable oils containing unsaturated fatty acids should be used as well as animal fats. Cod liver oil and halibut liver oils are also a useful adjunct to these diets.

Fish

Fish is as good, if not better than meat as a high protein exclusive diet and can be used in exactly the same way as that described for meat. The fish should be boiled and never fried. Cod, haddock, whiting, etc. are better than flat fish for this purpose. Only one warning—do not prolong an all-fish diet especially if warm water is used in place of fruit juices for the liquid. A long period exclusively on fish can be harmful but not at all if carried out only for periods mentioned here.

Naturopathy and Vegetarianism

The foregoing meat and fish diets have been set down as part of Naturopathic Practice in the knowledge that such diets will run counter to, and be resented by all avowed vegetarians. It is not intended in a book of this character to enter into any controversy regarding the rights and wrongs of an exclusively vegetarian diet. There are plenty of qualified champions to advocate the supposed rights and the wrongs of the vegetarian way of life. Naturopathy in itself is not synonymous with vegetarianism, and for this reason the instructions in this book enables both schools of thought to work out diets suited to the ethics of each. It is an old adage that "one man's meat is another man's poison" and it is certainly possible to work out a strictly vegetarian diet which will provide properly balanced nutrition for those whose principles preclude the eating of flesh foods. On the other hand, all the founders of Nature Cure implied a meat diet in their writings and many included, as here, all-meat and fish diets for use in certain cases.

It is sometimes maintained that the vegetarian life offers the chance of greater longevity, but there is little proof of this from statistics and vegetarians do not seem to enjoy any greater life span than meat eaters.

The protagonists for vegetarianism state that the elephant is a vegetarian and is one of the longest living mammals and that the parrot among the birds is long living and a vegetarian. Certainly this may be true but the parrot and the elephant are constructed by nature to be definite vegetarians just as are the cow and the horse, but neither of the latter could be said to enjoy any measure of longevity. At the same time, their teeth formations and digestive systems are very different from ours.

We maintain that anatomically and physiologically man is intended to be omniverous. We are not exclusively carnivorous, nor are we exclusively herbivorous. In other words, we may need meat and fish in our diet as well as fruits, vegetables and herbs, and we are equipped physically to deal equally with either form of food.

If, on the other hand, the deep conviction is held that for ethical or other reasons, an exclusively vegetarian diet should be adhered to, then the material in this book will help anyone with these convictions to work out the best possible diet to suit these circumstances and to ensure that in so doing a proper balance of nutrients is obtained. The pitfall of omitting essential and vital nutrients will be avoided as far as possible despite the restrictions imposed by confining the source of all foods to vegetable products. This does not apply in the case of vegans (those who also preclude all dairy produce from the diet). The present state of our knowledge of the preparation and manufacture of foods is such that it is impossible to supply complete and adequate nutrition, at the same time avoiding the use of all dairy products. As stated earlier, the day may not be far distant when we are able to extract from plants the first class protein said to be locked up in the cellulose of their structure and which in their present edible state are entirely unavailable to humans owing to the inability of our digestive systems to deal with them, and to release these proteins. It could well be that the ideals for which the vegetarian movement fights could be an accomplished fact overnight were the money now used in the development of atomic warfare for our own destruction used for the commercial production of plant protein for the common use and good. Until then it is felt necessary to include meat and fish in the diets of most of us, especially those engaged in manual labour and those who eat out and have difficulty in choosing at all times the best possible foods on which to live.

It is hoped that this explanation of our standpoint with regard to the use of flesh foods in therapeutic diets will not offend our vegetarian readers, but that they, like ourselves, will preserve a tolerant attitude to all points of view and use their own discretion in deciding, all things considered, which will be the diet most suited to themselves. This is the duty of each one of us. As previously stated, this book is intended to stimulate individual and rational thought on these matters rather than lay down any preconceived ideology to be blindly followed by the reader.

Unfired Foods

It is also necessary to mention another minority belief that only uncooked food is of any real value to man and that man was never intended to eat cooked food. However true this theory may be, it is also true that man has been eating cooked food for many thousands of years—and it is equally true that man, like some of the microbes we have dealt with, is a very adaptable and resistant creature. He has undoubtedly adapted himself to cooked foods for a very long time BUT also he has not lost the ability to eat raw foods. In other words, both cooked and unfired foods can have their place in the diet of any healthy human being, and we think that to endeavour to go back to an exclusively unfired diet would tax man's energies once again so that over generations he would have to re-adapt himself to this type of diet with consequent suffering in the meantime. Any adaptation to new environment or new ways of life is a form of evolution and cannot be carried out by nature for the many without the sacrifice in the process of the few. For this reason we do not give a clarion call of Back to Nature and the all-raw diet to those who wish in this lifetime to try and achieve a modicum of health and a continuity of vitality which is all too often absent because of ignorance of these very facts.

Quantitative Diet

We have dealt rather fully with the quality of our diet but there is another factor with which we should deal. This is—how much should we eat each day when we are healthy in order to maintain health without either overburdening the body or giving it too little food? This aspect of human nutrition is usually not mentioned in naturopathic text books, being left to the individual inclination and appetite. This in the case of a healthy man with a natural appetite is all very well, but we are trying to deal with cases which as a result of disease, are not healthy and which do not have healthy appetites in consequence—either physical or mental.

This is a difficult problem at best and here we endeavour to give a rough guide as to quantity which is considered most suitable for our own temperate climate. On the other hand, these instructions are subject to great variations in individual cases.

The average weight of the daily intake of food for the healthy adult should be about 3 to 4 lb. weight per day varying of course according to the type of work undertaken during the day. This should be split as follows: 1 lb. to $1\frac{1}{2}$ lb. of protein per day. 1 lb. to $1\frac{1}{2}$ lb. of fresh fruit per day and about $\frac{1}{2}$ lb. fresh vegetables with not more than $\frac{1}{2}$ lb. of whole grain cereal products.

The ideal during the summer months is protein and fresh fruit with green vegetable salads, while during the winter months carbohydrates in the form of cereals and starchy vegetables and fruits—more potatoes, bananas, etc., may be included. Naturally, we include with the protein and fruit during the summer a certain amount of fats and oils in the form of dried, sweet oily fruits and nuts. These will provide all we need by way of calories in addition to what we obtain from the protein, for as we know from previous chapters, protein will supply heat to the body and give us energy as well as many things which the exclusively energy-producing foods will not.

Now to the average weight of the healthy man. It is not easy to lay down hard and fast rules for, congenitally, men vary in their individual make-up, weight of bone structure, natural amount of covering flesh, etc. But for a good average, the following can be taken as a guide :

MALE : Age between 14 and 20, height 5 ft. 3 in.—120 lb. Same age with a height of 5 ft. 5 in. would be approx 128 lb.

Age between 20 and 30 with height 5 ft. 3 in.—124 lb. The same age group with height of 5 ft. 10 in. would be between 150 and 160 lb. and so on. The older age groups of the same heights would be relatively a little heavier. Details of average weights for age and heights can be obtained easily enough so only a rough outline is mentioned here.

FEMALES : They are, usually, for the same age and height, a few pounds lighter than their male counterparts.

This chapter concludes the section of our book dealing with dietetics and, if a thorough knowledge of this has been gained, the reader is in a position to use his own intelligence in arranging suitable diets to suit any eventuality.

When faced with a seemingly impossible task in respect of diet—try and take an objective look at the case. Forget the systems and methods you have already tried and tackle the problem anew. You may find that you have completely forgotten some small factor which will provide you with a clue as to the best possible therapy to employ, a clue which could turn out to be important enough to make a change of approach desirable. The secret of cure for any particular patient may well lie here.

Perseverence is the real secret of success, no matter to what school of healing a practitioner may belong. It is necessary to bring a singleness of purpose to bear on all problems which present themselves and to concentrate solely on this until it is satisfactorily solved. All good practitioners do this. They never give up themselves and they never let the patient give up—for this means defeat.

In the following chapter we commence the study of the next important branch in Naturopathic Practice—Hydrotherapy. This more than any other therapy is the complement of Dietetics. Water and earth, the cardinal elements of our own planet—our immediate surroundings—Diet and Hydrotherapy—these are a pair intimately connected with each other both as internal and external treatments. The other two cardinal elements, SUN and AIR, are of a higher order.

PART 3

HYDROTHERAPY

CHAPTER 15

WATER: INTERNAL AND EXTERNAL

Hydrotherapy is the natural treatment of disease by the application of water internally and externally in various forms and at different temperatures. It is a very powerful and effective form of treatment and usually readily available. It should be widely used as a natural form of healing in every naturopathic consulting room and clinic. The old saying of "familiarity breeds contempt" is particularly true in respect of the use of water as a healing agent. It is so cheap and easily obtained in climates like our own that it tends to be ignored, or if used, then in such a half-hearted and general manner as to not be specifically effective when it is needed most. It does appear that the majority would rather support the vested interests of the ointment manufacturers than go to the trouble of making and applying a simple water compress themselves. Perhaps it is the psychological aspect which has the effect of making anything which has to be paid for a better and more effective treatment than something that can be obtained very cheaply but in which there is an element of trouble in the preparation before the application can be made.

Conditions of Treatment

However this may be, it is quite certain that if water compresses were used in 95 per cent of the cases which resort to suppressive ointment, the results would in the end be far more spectacular and there would be a general emancipation resu.ting in a steady decline in the chemists' business.

In all cases of weak circulation, sluggish or inactive skin, eczemas, etc., and in fact in most cases of chronic disease such as deep-seated miasms, water treatment of the appropriate kind will be found of great value. It is a pity that in so many cases our various forms of Natural Therapeutics are so one-sided or are used by practitioners in a one-sided manner. Some will follow fasting and diet only with almost religious fanaticism, while others will practise the Schroth Cure exclusively, while yet others will practise the biochemic or homoeopathic systems to the exclusion of all other natural treatments. Natural therapy ceases to be effective as such when used in this way as it is only by the application of every possible indicated therapy that a real cure can result. Water treatment tends to be the poor relation of Naturopathy and in recent years has declined in use outside the Naturopathic Hydros. Our spas which were once so popular are now decaying relics of a past era—not because they were found wanting in efficacy but because today in the rush and turmoil of modern living there is no time to stay and undergo treatment properly. It is thought that suppressive drugs and applications will do the work of the spas far more quickly and effectively. Perhaps the symptoms are suppressed more quickly but are people really any better in health as a result— what about the ever-increasing incidence of heart disease, psycho-somatic complaints and the ever-growing army of chronic sufferers? It is little use cutting down the infantile death rate or extending the length of actual life if the period between birth and death is to be one long battle against chronic disease.

Father Kneipp

The pioneer of Hydrotherapy was undoubtedly Father Kneipp, and those readers who would wish to make a special study of this very fine system of healing would do well to obtain a copy of Kneipp's original work "Mein Wasser Kur" published in English by William Blackwood & Sons.

Father Kneipp, in addition to being the founder of Hydrotherapy as we know it today, was also an experienced herbalist and utilized all the folk herbs of Germany in his treatments, often using them in decoction and infusion form to be incorporated in packs and compresses as well as in hot baths. He is another great Naturopath who used herbal remedies extensively in his work. He maintained that water treatments achieved all the benefits of drug treatments in acute conditions without the after-toxinous or side effects. These treatments will relieve internal congestion and general internal heat, thus bringing about a dispersal of inflammation. Body temperature can be reduced below danger point by stimulating the radiation of heat through the skin. These are principles which must always be borne in mind when using hydrotherapy. The success of the treatment depends on the skill which is used in selecting the correct form it shall take. This is the real art of healing. Success will always depend on the ability to adopt the best type of treatment, bearing in mind the various pathological conditions as well as the symptoms. Also very important is to take into consideration the type of individual who is to undergo the treatment. People are not just a collection of parts or symptoms but whole thinking entities.

Water Temperatures

Never apply water to the body above 120° F. although the skin will tolerate a WATER VAPOUR temperature of around 140° F. and a dry air temperature of about 300° F.

Water temperatures from 32 to 45° F. are considered very cold while from 40 to 70° F. are considered from cold to cool and 80 to 95° F. are regarded as tepid to warm. The higher temperatures from 95 to 105° F. and higher are hot to very hot.

All baths of the warm variety are usually sedative in effect, especially if they are carried on for some time. On the other hand, the cold baths are stimulating when prescribed for short periods but can be depressing and not very helpful if they are too prolonged. The most stimulating effects are obtained from alternating hot and cold applications or baths.

Period and Effect

Very hot water for short periods will decrease the activity of the skin and lower the body temperature while stimulating the nervous system. It will strengthen the heart action and cause muscle contractions to stimulate breathing. Very hot treatments over a long time will increase the activity of the skin and raise the body temperature while lowering blood pressure. The heart will be weakened in its action and the muscles will be relaxed with dilation of the blood vessels. The whole metabolism is stimulated with quickened and weakened breathing.

Cold treatments are nearly always applied for short periods only and these increase the activity of the skin and raise the body temperature while stimulating the nervous system and strengthening the action of the heart. Metabolism is also stimulated and muscles and blood vessels are contracted for a short time. The breathing is slowed down and made deeper.

Types of Treatment

Water treatments can be local or general; internal or external. Local applications in the form of jets or packs have a generally local effect while general applications such as a complete body pack, steam room treatment or general baths have a general effect on the body.

For example, a very hot jet applied over the whole length of the spine, or alternatively a very hot pack, would lower blood pressure, while the same applications carried out with cold water would raise the blood pressure. A long hot application in the form of a pack over the heart would increase action and weaken the heart itself, while a prolonged cold application over the same organ would lessen its beat and give strength.

Local hot applications applied over long periods will soothe and relieve pain.

Hydrotherapy should always be commenced with short mild applications, gradually extending the time and going to the more extreme temperatures as the treatments proceed and the patient's toleration is extended.

Internal Water Treatments

These can be applied in varied ways and include the use of gravity douches, enemas, eye baths, mouth treatments, etc. Many of these are carried out with herbal infusions to increase the therapeutic effect and we shall deal with these at greater length later on.

The Epsom Salts Bath

This has long been a very popular form of hydrotherapeutic treatment, and although it is not herbal and makes use of a mineral salt, magnesium sulphate, it is a most effective way of increasing elimination of toxins and poisons from the system, particularly when these are caused by the various rheumatic diseases. They give immense relief in all cases of muscular pain and all cases of chronic rheumatism should benefit from the regular use of them. It usually takes the form of a complete bath. $3\frac{1}{2}$ lb. of commercial epsom salts (obtainable from most chemists at a reasonable price in 7 lb. bags) are dissolved in a bath of very hot water and the patient is instructed to lie completely immersed (except for the head) for five minutes. Vigorous drying follows with a rough towel, and the patient then rests for an hour or more so that the therapeutic effect which continues after the bath, shall not be impeded. These baths are usually taken once weekly, and each succeeding bath is increased in length until a maximum of twenty minutes is reached. It will be found that even after the first bath, most inflammatory rheumatic conditions will respond and provide considerable relief from pain and other adverse symptoms. At the same time a good progressive internal herbal treatment with correct diet should be established. In the rheumatic cases where loss of mobilization has been experienced in joints, these baths can be the prelude to good massage and soft tissue manipulations when mobility can be restored after the acute inflammatory stages of the disease have passed.

Epsom salts can also be used locally in packs and compresses either hot or cold. These are particularly useful where joints are inflamed and there is restriction of movement. The cold compress will be found best and this is usually left on overnight. A piece of sheeting just large enough to cover the area is soaked in the cold epsom salts solution (about $\frac{1}{4}$ lb. of the salts to half a pint of water). Wring out not quite dry and place over the area or joint. Wrap this up carefully with some old woolly garment and loosely bind in place. The patient should be told that if the sensation of relief and warmth is produced during the first twenty minutes (and this often happens in a very few minutes), the compress should be left on all night. If no heat is generated, it should be taken off and a further effort made with a cold compress after frequent warm applications. Usually the cold compress will be found to work first time. These compresses should be applied for three consecutive nights and left off for the same time and then repeated. Soap must never be used with any epsom salt treatments as this will destroy the therapeutic action of the magnesium sulphate.

Sauna or Steam Baths

Only a brief mention need be made here of steam baths which are readily obtainable in most large cities. Regretfully, they are much more popular on the Continent than in the United Kingdom. Sometimes they are called Russian baths. Home steam cabinets can also be bought at quite reasonable prices.

The Turkish bath is the hot dry heat bath, and the suana is more dry than the Russian or Wet Steam bath which is made by injecting jets of steam into a special room at varying temperatures. The jets can be medicated with herbal aromatics such as pine, menthol, mint, etc., for the treatment of bronchitis. In many specially constructed establishments, the Turkish and Russian bath can be taken together and the prices of such treatments, when local council operated, are very reasonable indeed. These amenities, furnished out of local rates, are not usually appreciated by the mass of ratepayers and "addicts" are usually tired business men wishing to reduce weight caused by lack of exercise and over-indulgence and those few who really appreciate the value of such treatments in keeping fit. Short spells in the steam room alternated with strong, cold jet showers, are immensely stimulating and very good for general health and for the skin in particular. It must be borne in mind, however, that these baths should not be taken too frequently and one fortnightly or monthly is quite enough for general health purposes as distinct from using them as a therapy in the treatment of some particular condition.

An important point to remember:— if it is desired to accentuate the effect of the hot steam, a glass of COLD water should be taken immediately prior to going into the steam room. Heavy meals should never be taken before these baths and it is always best to let a couple of hours elapse after a meal before taking a steam or Turkish bath.

The medicated variety are also extremely beneficial for acute head colds, bronchitis and blocked nasal passages as well as in the more chronic conditions of the respiratory tract. At home the same effect can be obtained locally by holding the head over a large basin of boiling water covered with a towel and inhaling the steam either plain or with the water suitably infused with a good herbal such as elder flowers, mint or both.

Hot Baths

The straightforward hot bath is a powerful stimulant to elimination. The skin, being one of the organs of elimination is the one most affected. Tension and congestion is relieved and the body is able to throw off accumulations of toxins and waste. In doing this the kidneys are assisted and relieved in their function and in general the results of overstrain such as stiffness and soreness of muscles and joints is instantly relieved. They are best taken immediately before retiring like the epsom salts bath and whenever possible, in the case of the plain hot bath, a shower of the same temperature should follow to cleanse the body before drying and retiring. Kidney disease, catarrhal infections, rheumatism, skin eruptions, neuritis and many other complaints are benefited by the hot bath—and what a simple remedy and one which can be undertaken in almost any home. It is a "must" for all athletes after exercise. A variation for athletes can be taken in shower form—a very hot shower followed by a very cold one of very short duration. The whole organism is then completely refreshed and re-invigorated. Hot baths should not be taken too frequently, once weekly or fortnightly is quite often enough.

Warm Baths

These can be taken daily and are most valuable in chronic skin affections, convulsions, spasms of all kinds and in disease of the genito-urinary system. The duration of these baths can be up to one hour or even longer if required.

Cool Baths

These are of most use in cases of the elderly and the very infirm in place of the cold bath. The practitioner will make up his mind on examination which kind of bath the patient will be most fitted for. It is a matter of general common-sense deciding which temperature is most suited to individual needs. In any case, is is always good practice to commence with the more moderate type of bath and proceed to the extremes as the treatment gets under way. No shock and unnecessary pain is then caused to the patient but a feeling of some progress is felt from the commencement, no matter how slow it may appear.

Cold Baths

These are best taken when the body has been thoroughly warmed so that the reaction is complete. Then only is the best tonic effect obtained. The entire body is stimulated and a feeling of well-being suffuses the system. They should be of short duration and never more than five minutes, after which the body is vigorously rubbed down. A very cold bath should never exceed one or two minutes followed by a rub down with strong rough towelling. The average for this type of bath is once daily except in hot climates where more than one cold shower may be taken during the day with no ill effects.

Soap and Baths

Before leaving the subject of baths, mention should be made

of cleansing baths, using soap as the cleansing agent. This type of bath is known to everyone. It should not be taken more than twice weekly or perhaps three times according to the type of work in which the patient is involved.

It is well-known that the skin, apart from being an eliminative organ, is also a secondary breathing organ, and for this reason the pores of the skin should always be kept clean and open. Soap is not always the ideal means of doing this, and soap scum left on the skin can have an adverse effect on general health, placing a larger burden than necessary on the lungs. This is more particularly true when there is a tendency to bronchitis or other respiratory infection. It is really essential to have a hot shower followed by a tepid rinse after a soap bath. The skin also secretes natural oils and other substances which can be destroyed by the too frequent use of soap. The skin will then dry up giving the appearance of premature old age. Never wash the face with soap and water more than once daily. The face is the most exposed part of the body and will "weather" very quickly if a lot of soap is used, thereby destroying the natural oils and leaving the face unprotected against winds and extreme weather conditions generally.

This general survey of complete body baths provides a knowledge of the conditions for which they are best suited and under what circumstances it is best to apply them—the effects of the different bath temperatures and the diseases in which they will be found most effective. The actual metabolic and physiological effects of various baths are given, which will enable the reader to work out a suitable water treatment for any condition including the most general ones stated. In the next chapter the use of specific compresses and packs will be investigated in order to make this section on Hydrotherapy as complete as possible.

CHAPTER 16

THE WATER JET

The water jet was mentioned in the last chapter in conjunction with general body baths. It is sometimes called a douche bath and can be used alone and for the same purpose as the general body bath. The temperatures will be chosen in the same way as for the general body bath. It is perhaps the most powerful form of hydrotherapy and can be used internally as well as externally in appropriate pressures for the nose, ear, stomach, rectum, bladder, vagina and urethra.

Most health homes are fitted with a variety of types of these douches or jets and some of the less expensive ones are also very practical for use in the private house.

Epsom salts is not the only addition to the water bath and douche which is widely used. The various local douche treatments for the ear, eye, nose, etc., can have herbal additives which are of great practical help just as the general bath can, instead of magnesium sulphate, have the addition of seaweed, salt, sea salt, and many herbals. Some brief indications of the best uses of these will be given later in this chapter.

The Sitz Bath

This is intended as a treatment for the pelvic region and is valuable in all cases of haemorrhoids, disorders of the reproductive organs such as impotence, sciatica, lumbago and all the other forms of lower back strain and sprain which are so common. The temperature is always chosen by taking into account the general physical condition of the patient and virtually the same rules apply as have been outlined for the general baths. They are useful as a treatment for prolapse in women.

The Whole Body Pack—the Schroth True Wet Pack Treatment

The whole body pack or wet sheet pack as it is also called,

encloses the entire body and is ideal, in conjunction with fasting, for all types of inflammation, fevers and metabolic disturbances. It is also known as the sweat pack.

It should only ever be given in a properly heated room. It is best to keep a bed specially for this purpose. The bedclothes are rolled back and a thick blanket is spread over the bottom bed sheet (to keep the bed sheet dry, a second blanket may be laid beneath the pack blanket). A sheet measuring about 6 ft. × 5 ft. of unbleached cotton twill is wrung out in cold water. The result should not be too wet and not too dry. Do not have it dripping water but at the same time it must not be fully wrung out. This is now spread over the pack blanket and the patient, completely nude, is placed reclining backwards on the sheet, which is then wrapped round the whole body excluding the arms and head only. The feet should be kept apart at least a foot. The blanket is then wrapped over the sheet and the whole secured with clips and safety pins so that the result appears rather like a sleeping bag. A further blanket of thick wool can be placed over the whole in the usual way. The patient remains in this pack from three to eight hours and when taken out a cold sponge is applied and the patient completely sponged down before being dried with a good rough towel. After this the patient is transferred to a warm dry bed for complete rest and relaxation for another hour or two.

The Local Wet Pack

This is of most value in helping to reduce local swellings and inflammations. Here the pack is used over the actual area affected, as well as the immediately adjacent parts. If, for example, the wrist is swollen and inflamed, use the local pack on the entire arm. Use a piece of old sheeting and wring out in water, again leaving it not too wet and not too dry, and using just enough material to cover the area required, in this case the arm. Wrap round the arm but without allowing any restriction of movement. Always make sure that any compress or pack is comfortable. Cover this with warm woollen material and secure with clips or pins. A feeling of warmth should be experienced in about five to ten minutes—if not it should be removed and heat applied before a further trial is made of the cold pack. A pack of this kind is left on for anything from two hours to all night. It is a good plan when these are used to make a point of applying them just before going to bed and when they prove effective, leave them on all night. Always apply a cold sponge wash to the parts after a local pack and then dry thoroughly. They can be applied for three nights in succession and then left off for three nights, repeating until the inflammation has entirely disappeared.

An abdominal pack should be made large enough to cover the hips, reaching well above and below. It is very successful in arthritis of the hip joint and again is most effective when carried out just before retiring. Hot water bottles can be placed at the outside of the pack against the thighs to increase the effect of the pack and ensure warmth of the surroundings. The hot water bottles are especially useful in the case of old people and those of poor vitality generally.

The value of these packs in the treatment of rheumatic joints will be greatly increased if nettles or elder flowers are used and the packs can also be alternated with applications of ointments of the herbal kind like thuja or chickweed. Chickweed is extremely valuable for sore and swollen feet. In using nettles, elder flowers or other herbal infusions, make the infusion first, using about a pound of the dried herb to a pint of water. Chill in a fridge before straining for use in the pack.

A cold pack will often serve to prevent the formation of an abscess in appendicitis whereas hot water applications or hot water bottles may well commence the formation of an abscess. Of course appendicitis, like many other complaints, will also require internal treatment and homoeopaths have found that iris tenax 12x given internally is almost a specific in cases of acute appendicitis.

Colonic Irrigation

In all cases of long standing and chronic disease, as well as the more obvious conditions of constipation, the patient should commence naturopathic treatment with a course of colonic irrigations, either while fasting or on a restricted diet. It is amazing how often sufferers hitherto listless and without any energy take on a new lease of life after a course of colonic irrigations.

It has been said that this is not in fact a natural treatment at all but most certainly a very good example of its use in nature can be cited. The ibis is a bird which travels very long distances over desert country and as so often happens in such parts, arrives at an oasis practically exhausted. The ibis does not, like the human, immediately drink its fill of water on arrival. Oh no! Its first task it to give itself an enema. It is very well equipped to do this on account of its long bill and it obviously knows instinctively that an irrigation will reduce the exhaustion and revive the metabolism far better than taking a long drink of water first. In this way the long dehydrating experience of a long flight across the desert is overcome in the shortest possible time.

Anyone wishing to take a colonic irrigation should always be properly prepared by spending at least one day on an all-fruit diet before taking the irrigation. At least eight hours should have elapsed after the last fruit meal and it is always best done after a night's rest.

The gravity douche is the most natural way of doing this. The special apparatus installed in many Nature Cure Homes is very commendable but not practicable in the private house and results with the gravity douche can be just as good. They can be obtained at most chemists in various capacity sizes at a very reasonable cost. It is best to obtain an 8 pint size as this can then be used for lesser amounts when required, while 8 pints is the normal maximum ever taken in this way.

The first irrigation should not exceed one pint of water at body temperature and this amount can be increased by a half pint to a pint each succeeding day until the patient's maximum has been reached. If a complete course of douches is not being taken, a general douche of about two pints is used.

The patient is placed in position before the container is filled in order to prevent the water being cooled to any degree before it is taken. Two positions are favoured for the introduction of the water. The first, and perhaps the best position, is to have the patient lying on the left side. The second position is in a kneeling or crouching position. NEVER HAVE THE PATIENT LYING ON THE RIGHT SIDE. The nozzle of the irrigator is lubricated with vaseline and after making sure that there is no air in the apparatus, it is inserted in the rectum and the water released by the clip supplied. It should flow smoothly into the colon. When the desired amount of water has been absorbed, the patient should continue to lie on the left side for ten minutes and then turn to lie on the back for a further ten minutes. While in this position the abdomen can be carefully and gently kneaded so as to give every opportunity for the loosening of dry hard matter and impacted faeces which may be lodged on the walls of the colon. After this the patient again turns over to the other side for another ten minutes, followed by ten minutes in the face down or prone position. If, during this time the retention of the water becomes intolerable, then it should be expelled and a longer time aimed at with the next irrigation.

If it is found impossible to hold the water for this length of time on the first day, there is no cause for alarm and greater lengths of time can be aimed at quite successfully in following treatments until a maximum of forty minutes has been reached. Quite often the crustations of many years will be harmlessly expelled by a course of these irrigations and in many cases the patient will literally feel rejuvenated.

The Value of Herbs

In colonic irrigations, as well as in the baths and packs, herbal infusions, as already stated, can be a great advantage. For example, in cases of colitis the addition of a fluid extract or an infusion of hydrastis (golden seal) is of great benefit. This will cleanse and tone up the membranes after they have been freed from the hardened waste of, in many cases, years standing. If the fluid extract is used, the proportion is one ounce of the extract to one pint of water. Infusions can be made as already described and the strained liquid heated to the required temperature. For piles and ruptured blood vessels, fluid extract of oak bark or witch hazel can be used in the same proportions.

Fluid extract of Saw Palmetto used in this way has been found to work wonders in cases of prostate gland inflammation in the male. In these cases, at the end of the usual course of irrigations described above, a rather stronger mixture of 2 oz. fluid extract of Saw Palmetto to one pint of water should be made and only one pint used. This is retained then for one or two hours for best results. Saw Palmetto can also be given as an internal treatment for this condition.

Epsom Salts Irrigation

Epsom salts is as useful and effective in irrigations as it is for baths and compresses. For irrigation purposes it is better to use the purified variety rather than the commercial type. The quantity usual for epsom salts is half an ounce to a pint of water. It can be used with every confidence in all toxic and rheumatic conditions.

Some exponents always insist on a fast during colonic irrigation treatment, but this is not always required and indeed in some deficiency diseases it is contra indicated. Fasting in conjunction with irrigations is always useful in the case of overweight sedentary workers, but fasting and colonic irrigation is NOT the panacea of all ills that some authorities would have us believe and it is this kind of claim which brings any treatment into disrepute.

Sea Salt

Useful in enemas and in baths. It has a wonderful tonic effect and is indicated in all cases of Bright's Disease and diabetes. Moistened sea salt can be rubbed over the entire body until a glow is effected and again has a tonic effect in the diseases mentioned.

Iodine

Another very useful ingredient for baths and compresses is in the form of KELP or SEAWEED. It can be added in quite substantial amounts to baths and the kelp can be made into mud compresses and packs for the skin—very useful in all the rheumatic inflammations of joints, etc.

Sulphur Baths

Flowers of sulphur can be added to baths with generally beneficial results in cases of tender skin, etc. A proportion of 2 oz. of Pot. sulphate to fifteen gallons of water is good in general bath treatments.

Pine Baths

For chest and lung affections, there is nothing like a pine needle bath. The needles should be gathered freshly fallen and added in large quantities. These with hydrastic colonic irrigations have helped many bronchitics.

Castor Oil Enema

In most cases of the elderly and those with weak constitutions, where there is a history of chronic constipation over long periods, it is advisable to precede a course of colonic irrigations with an enema of castor or olive oil.

This is done by injecting about six ounces of either oil as high as possible into the rectum and proceeding with irrigation of about one pint to one quart of water about half an hour afterwards. If a strong purgative is required, about 1 to $1\frac{1}{2}$ ounces of glycerine can be used. The oils or glycerine will, as in the case of irrigations, be at blood heat before use.

MOLASSES : between two and eight ounces of molasses stirred into one or two pints of water also makes an ideal purgative enema.

Stomach Lavage

Washing out the stomach is another useful aid to Naturopathic Practice and assists detoxication in many chronic disease conditions. This is done with the use of a length of suitable rubber tubing to which is attached a rubber or glass funnel.

The patient can either sit up in bed or in a chair with head bent slightly forward. The tube is placed into the back of the throat and the patient is asked to swallow while the tube is fed gently with a downward pressure of the tube. If there is any feeling on the part of the patient of choking, he should be told to take a long breath and say "AH". When the tube has reached the stomach, a pint of warm water is introduced slowly into the funnel and when this has all been taken, the funnel is lowered below the stomach level when the water will be syphoned out again. Repeat this process until the water syphoned away is clean and clear.

This treatment will remove accumulated mucous, acids and waste products, at the same time toning up the membrane and stomach lining. Hydrastis (Golden Seal) infusion or fluid extract added to the final lavage is an effective way of reducing inflammation.

From this study of the various kinds of water treatment, it will be seen that Hydrotherapy does form a very useful and extensive form of healing within the orbit of Naturopathic Practice. With a sound knowledge of this the reader is equipped to take advantage of water treatments whenever possible. Even the healthy will find pleasure in following many of the baths and jets for general tonic purposes. The sick and ailing will find them of inestimable use in their efforts to get back their health. Those in search of beauty will find that the inner cleanliness offered by colonic irrigations and supplemented by various herbal compresses according to the type of skin as facial packs, are far more valuable and effective than many of the spurious creams and patent face packs offered to the ladies today. There is no substitute for health and once obtained, this will radiate from and infuse the whole personality. It is something positive and dynamic. There is no easy way to its attainment especially in an age when mankind is beset on all sides with temptations which always seem to lead away from health.

We have now reached the stage when we have a knowledge of some of the natural therapies and are able to carry out treatments in a safe and confident way. But in order that these treatments may be used in every case with the best possible effect, it is necessary to know something of pathology and what happens when the various structures of the body undergo change resulting from disease. In the next chapters, this subject and the methods used to arrive at an accurate picture of the patient's condition, will be explained.

PART 4

PATHOLOGY AND DIAGNOSIS

CHAPTER 17

PATHOLOGY

Chemical, functional and structural changes which occur during disease are known as pathological changes. These changes vary in degree and extent of severity according to the length and chronicity of the disease. It is the scientific observation of these pathological changes which help the practitioner to decide on treatment and to vary this according to the changes which take place or are prompted by the treatment undertaken.

In order to have a sound knowledge of pathology, it is first essential to know something of cell structure in its healthy state. Every living organism is made up of one or many cells according to the complexity of the organism. There are forms of single cellular life such as amoebae. In the case of this tiny animal the whole of the life functions are carried out by a single cell. In the case of some of the most complex forms of organism such as man, we find that certain cells combine together to form specialized organs with each organ forming some part of his life. In a sense these organs have and lead separate lives and the health of an individual man depends on the health of the individual cells which make up the individual organs and structures of the body. The ultimate health of the man depends on the harmony with which the several parts or separate organs work together and each organ depends for its health on the health of the individual cells of which it is composed.

Individual Cells

There are cells of all sizes and shapes. There are polyhedral cells, round, oval and spindle-shaped cells as well as cells of irregular shape. It is a fact that cells of any particular organ or structure strongly resemble all other cells of that organ with which they are so closely associated. In other words, although there is an almost infinite variety of cells, those having the same or similar functions are similar in external appearance.

A cell can be examined under a microscope. Each individual cell is encapsulated by a membrane or cell wall which forms a protection. This in the case of animal cells is called by the general name of plasma membrane. As we shall not be dealing with plant cells, it is sufficient to remark that vegetable or plant cells are made of cellulose and are very freely permeable. The cell wall in man is not composed of cellulose but of varying living substances which are not freely permeable but only selectively so. The varying degree of selectivity is due to the varying chemical composition of the cell walls, and it can be affected by the chemical compounds which may be surrounding the cell.

The viscid, colourless and almost transparent substance which forms the interior of the cell is known as protoplasm. Again, there are many form or types of protoplasm. This fluid surrounds a thread-like network which is believed to be the living part of the cell while the fluid supplies nutrition to and activates the cell. The living network of the cell is known as the spongioplasm and the fluid which surrounds it is called hyoplasm.

In each cell is a small mass of highly differentiated protoplasm which is called the nucleus and is the centre of the cell life's activity. It is responsible for the whole life of the cell and cells of course have different kinds of work to do in a complex structure such as the human body. Some have the job of absorbing foreign and diseased substances and have more than one nucleus. They are called giant cells.

Leucocyte Cells

This is a colourless amoeboid cell with a highly specialized job for which purpose it is able to move about the body from place to place. It absorbs waste matter and foreign substances to fight disease. The white blood corpuscles are examples of leucocyte although there are other leucocytes besides these. Each nucleus has its own membrane within which is its own NUCLEAR NETWORK, known as ACHROMATIN. Without a nucleus a cell is dead although it can carry on certain destructive and neutral processes. It can never carry on any constructive process and it can never reproduce itself.

Functions

As the cells of the body have specialized functions in groups making up organs and other structures, they can under certain abnormal influences and conditions also take on other functions. For example, the ENDOTHELIAL CELLS or those lining serous cavities, lymphatics, blood vessels and liver and kidneys can become PHAGOCYTES. That is, they will possess the property of ingesting and digesting bacteria and fragments of morbid matter or other cells.

Cell Reproduction

Growth in man and animals depends on cells multiplying. The term used to define cell reproduction in a general sense is KARYOKINESIS and it covers two main methods of cell subdivision. Cells can subdivide by means of the nucleus of the cell contracting and separating by direct fission. When this happens, the main body of the cell follows suit and the result is two cells. This process is then repeated in each of the two new cells and so on. This process is known as DIRECT CELL DIVISION or AMITOSIS. The other method of cell division is known as MITOSIS and this method differs from AMITOSIS in that a gradual and continuous process of change takes place in the nucleus and cytoplasm. This method of INDIRECT CELL DIVISION is caused by gradual changes in the chromatin network of the nucleus, both chemical and physical, and the centrosomes move away from each other and establish their own spheres of attraction (centrosphere).

Pathological Cell Division. It is possible that when the splitting of the chromatic threads on division is unequal, one of the resultant nucleii has a larger number of these bodies than the other. The one with too few is called a hypochromatic nucleus and that with too many is a hyperchromatic necleus. This kind of division is pathological and can be seen in some manifestations of cancer. In some cases when the cell divides, the spindle produces more than two poles, we have multipolar mitrosis and this condition again occurs in some kinds of cancer cells.

Cell Uses

Cells generally may be classified into three groups—those of GROWTH, *Maintenance* and *Reproduction* and those with some special function. Cell activity continues throughout life. If any of these functions ceases, degenerative changes take place and we have what we call a pathological condition. Like every other form of life, cells can only continue to live while they can adapt themselves to changing conditions of environment, etc. Changes can be brought about by external conditions such as pressures, burns, etc. If these changes are such that the cell cannot adapt itself, then pathology will result. Internal changes can be brought about in the blood or lymph and these will affect the various organs. Endocrine glands can be affected so as to impair the amount of hormone secreted. This can result in hormone deficiency, and if the cells involved cannot correct it, a pathological condition will result. Various biochemical substances may occur in too large or too small quantities and thus interfere with the life of the cell and again produce a pathological change by interfering with the proper function of the cell or cells involved. A functional change in an organ can also account for abnormal constituents being produced either as secretions or excretions. In the case of the kidneys, abnormal constituents can be found in the urine. As another example, if the left ventricle, as in cases of chronic mitral stenosis, becomes poorly supplied with blood, the tissue will become atrophied. All the ordinary physiological changes which take place under normal conditions can, in certain circumstances, become modified so as to produce abnormal and pathological results.

If a cell absorbs too much lymph fluid, the supporting networks become cloudy, swell and break down. Vacuoles are formed which increase in size and number until the whole structure disintegrates and dies. These are known as cytoplasmic changes. In cases where the nucleus itself breaks down and becomes fragmented, the chromatin is distributed throughout the cell. This kind of degeneration is known as KARYORRHEXIS.

Classification of Disease

From this very (and necessarily brief) survey, the student will at once realize that the health of the whole body is ultimately dependent on the health of each individual cell and the sum total of health will only equal the harmony and health of the cells which make up the entire body structure of man.

The results of these pathological changes are disease in the individual and this can be acute or chronic. In addition to acute and chronic disease which most students will already be acquainted with, there are many other classifications and we list some here :

CONGENITAL. Disease present at birth.

CONSTITUTIONAL. Affecting the metabolism.

CONTAGIOUS. Caught by contact.

DEFICIENCY. Resulting from defective metabolism and due to lack of essential nutrients, e.g., vitamins, trace elements, etc.

DIFFUSE. Attacking several or all of the spinal cord tracts.

DYNAMIC. Functional.

ENDEMIC. Recurring or continuous in a particular part.

EPIDEMIC. Attacking large numbers in the same locale.

FUNCTIONAL. Disease in which there are no apparent anatomical lesions to account for it.

HEREDITY. Transmitted from parent to child from one generation to another.

IDIOPATHIC. Disease for which there is no apparent cause.

INFECTIOUS. Caused by micro-organisms either airborne or water-borne. This type of disease does not have to be the result of contact with an infected person.

INTERSTITIAL. Where connective tissue or the framework of organs is involved.

ORGANIC. Where there is degenerative anatomical changes in tissue or organs.

PANDEMIC. Disease which is known throughout the world.

PERIODIC. Disease recurring at definite intervals.

SPECIFIC. Produced by a special micro-organism.

SPORADIC. Disease which occurs in isolated cases and is neither endemic nor epidemic.

SUBACUTE or SUBCHRONIC. CONDITIONS WHICH ARE BETWEEN CHRONIC AND ACUTE.

ZYMOTIC. Disease of an infectious nature resulting from the action of a living ferment (zymase).

Survey of Pathological Conditions

We list now a short survey of the pathological conditions which are most usually encountered in various forms of disease. It must be realized, however, that there are many others and some which are incapable of being observed or recorded. Much work is still being carried out by research laboratories on pathological changes which take place in the human body. It is the practitioner's duty to keep abreast of modern findings. Never be prejudiced by the source of the knowledge for all schools of healing can contribute in this field.

The list which follows is as far as possible in alphabetical order only :

1. ABSCESS. This is the formation of pus in a cavity on or near the body surface. It is a local condition. When there is a collection of pus in the same way in a cavity of the body it is called EMPYEMA.

2. ANAEMIA. This is a condition where the proportion of red blood corpuscles to white is diminished and the quantity of blood is lessened.

3. ATROPHY. This is a condition in which wasting and shrinkage occur, resulting in the decrease in size of an organ or part.

4. CANCER. This is a general term really as there are two categories of cancer, namely CARCINOMA and SARCOMA. CARCINOMA is made up of a malignant tumour composed of connective tissue enclosed by epithelial cells. When the enclosing membrane is broken or ruptured, the disease will spread rapidly. SARCOMA is a tumour consisting of a substance like the embryonic connective tissue and is not so localized as is carcinoma. Some of the pathological cell changes which occur have been described earlier.

5. CATARRHAL INFLAMMATION. This is an inflammatory condition of any mucous membrane. If there is suppuration, this is known as purulent, and when this happens to fibrous tissue it is known as fibrinous.

6. CYST. This is a non-malignant or benign form of tumour. Here the morbid matter is entirely enclosed in a sac. It can occur anywhere.

7. EDEMA. A swelling caused by infiltration of lymph or water from the blood vessels to the intercellular spaces or connective tissues.

8. EMBOLISM. Is a clot or obstruction which is carried round the blood vessels.

9. FEVER. This is a pathological condition where changes occur which raise the body temperature above normal.

10. FATTY DEGENERATION. This is a condition where normal body cells turn to fat.

11. GANGRENE. Is the decomposition of soft, living tissue of the body. There are two kinds, DRY and MOIST. The dry variety usually occurs in the superficial parts and is due to loss of nutrition due to restricted blood supply. The moist variety occurs in the deep-seated tissues where there is no evaporation. The cause is the same.

12. HYPERTROPHY. Is an increase in the size of tissues and cells and is the opposite to atrophy, caused by overwork of a part with increased blood supply.

13. HYPERPLASIA. Is the increase in the size of an organ or

part of the body brought about by the increase in the number of its component cells.

14. HYPERAEMIA. Is the increase in the amount of blood cells found in any organ or part of the body. This means either venous or arterial blood.

15. HAEMORRHAGE. This is a loss or escape of blood due to rupture of its containing vessel. If a tumour is formed of blood, it is called an hematonia.

16. ISCHAEMIA. This is the opposite of hyperaemia and describes a decrease in the amount of blood present in an organ or part of the body.

17. INFLAMMATION. This is a primary pathology and is caused by the effects of any kind of irritation on living tissue. It is a natural reaction whereby there is a rush of blood to the part affected, resulting in abnormal heat, swelling and consequent pain. Inflammation is described in many ways and takes many forms.

18. LEUKAEMIA. This is a condition in which there is an abnormal increase in the number of leukocytes in the blood. It is a form of cancer of the blood. Leukocytosis is another name for the same condition.

19. NECROSIS. Is the molecular or molar death of a tissue especially of the bone, while caries is the molecular death of bone structure, e.g., teeth.

20. THROMBOSIS. This is caused by the formation of or the presence of a thrombus in a blood vessel where it is formed. The thrombus itself is said to be caused by thrombin or thrombosin changing fibrinogen into fibrin.

Pathology is another science which helps the practitioner to build up a complete picture of the real condition of the individual. This is the basic condition of structural and chemical change taking place in component cells which underlie the symptomology experienced by the patient. In other words, the symptomology is the evidence of the presence of pathology which leads us to arrive at a proper diagnosis of the patient's condition.

CHAPTER 18

NATUROPATHY AND SYMPTOMOLOGY

Many schools of Naturopathy believe and teach that symptoms are not important, and that it is the underlying cause which is all that need concern the Naturopathic practitioner as it is causes which we cure, and not symptoms. They maintain that no useful purpose is served by a study of symptomology as all symptoms disappear when the cause of them is removed.

But, as any student of homoeopathy will know, the symptoms can be of very great importance to the practitioner as they are in fact the evidence which will lead him to suspect the real cause or pathological condition underlying them and thus help in formulating a correct diagnosis without which any sound or rational treatment would be impossible. From the homoeopathic point of view, it is only very careful observation of symptoms which will lead the practitioner to the correct similium (remedy) and for this reason the system of medicine known as Homoeopathy has much less need of pathology than it does of symptomology and homoeopathy is rightly a form of Naturopathic Practice but one which is a complete study in itself.

Etiology

From an evaluation of the symptomology, and pathological conditions which have produced it, the practitioner is often able to provide an ETIOLOGY of the disease from which a patient may be suffering. This is the REAL CAUSE OF THE DISEASE. For this the practitioner will also have to have the complete history of the patient if he is to provide good and effective treatment for the removal of the basic causes which gave rise to the pathological changes recorded by the symptomology.

There can, however, be some measure of agreement with some of the Naturopathic schools of thought mentioned and their teachings regarding the causative factors of disease. For often simple causes can be removed very effectively and certainly their removal will create an immediate improvement and early cure of the patient's condition. One such group of these causes may be termed environmental and in a loose way we can include the following causes which every practitioner should look for when obtaining the patient's history, etc. :

1. *Baths*—does the patient have the right kind of bath at the right time?
2. *Work*—what does he work at and what kind of things does he come in contact with?
3. *Exercise*—does he have regular and consistent exercise as distinct from a Saturday run around a football field to the exclusion of other better, more regular types of physical activity?
4. *Loss of light*—under what conditions does he live? Is his home and place of work properly lit? Does he have an adequate amount of sunshine and fresh air *every day*?
5. *Sleep*—under what conditions does he relax? Does he sleep under ideal conditions—room well aired, warm and fresh, etc.? Quite often even the direction of the patient's lying in bed will make a difference, for example lying head north and feet south is considered ideal.
6. *Clothing*—what kind of clothing does he wear? Is he coddled or too tightly clad? Does his clothing cause skin irritation or restriction of circulation, for example from tight elastic bands round the waist? Does the dye of clothes rub off on the skin? Investigate every aspect of clothing, dyes in fabrics, etc.
7. *Diet*—a great deal has already been said about the subject in these pages but this is such an important factor that it can never be emphasized too frequently. What kind of food has the patient been living on? Is it properly prepared and adequately balanced for his occupational needs? Does he have proper meal

times with enough time for proper mastication and digestion? Proper mental relaxation during the meal, etc.? What are the cooking utensils made of?

Co-ordination

It is only by a really thorough investigation into mode of life with an equally thorough investigation into the symptoms and pathology that real help and sound constructive advice can be given in every aspect of life that will affect individual health.

It is essential to co-ordinate the whole of the knowledge obtained about a patient and to make sure that it is as all-embracing as possible. From this, use can be made of all the indicated therapies outlined in this book as and when they are applicable so that the best possible results can be obtained from them. It is only in this way that anyone can be properly and completely cured and rehabilitated, with the least possible risk of a return of disease conditions.

Remember that if the complaint is to do with living conditions, food, clothes, housing, individual habits, etc., no lasting improvement will be possible unless and until these factors have been changed and improved in every respect. No avenue of environment or habit must be left unexplored in dealing with any ill person and if it is a matter of self-treatment, this will require a great deal of self-analysis carried out as impartially as possible, before treatment is commenced. Here the old adage of "Man know Thyself" (another Ancient Greek motto worthy of emulation) is of the greatest value. To be honest with oneself is to have half won any battle against disease.

Mental State

It is in this context that the mental state of a patient is so important and also has to be carefully observed in connection with everything else. Find out whether a mental condition is congenital or due to environnment or association with particular types which are incompatible with the personality being studied. Worries, emotions, tempers, grief and every other possible mental disturbance which could, however remotely, have a bearing on the case must be taken into consideration.

Excesses

Sexual excesses, eating to excess, etc., will also affect the health and mental outlook of each individual but appetites and requirements differ with individuals, for each human being is different from every other. Alcoholic indulgence must also be considered. Inhibitions, suppressions, repressions and in fact everything about a patient are of the deepest concern to any good Naturopath. The patient must always have the fullest confidence in his mentor and only the genuine ability and understanding of a practitioner will promote this confidence and make it justifiable to the extent that the fullest possible advantage can be obtained from any prescribed treatment.

Pots and Pans

Under item (7) the question—"what are the cooking utensils made of?" is asked. This is a very important point. Many practitioners are fully aware that patients who have displayed symptoms of chronic indigestion over long periods of time and who have not responded to treatment have made remarkable recoveries when it was found they were using aluminium for cooking and this was immediately stopped. It is very easy to overlook this point and so it is stressed here.

The more recent common use of stainless steel for the manufacture of cooking utensils has brought further hazards to health. Recent research carried out in the United States of America found that minute traces of chrome were liable to be absorbed by food cooked in this way and then taken as part of the diet. The effect of this is said to increase the incidence of heart disease and particularly of coronary thrombosis. These researchers also said that the only antidote to this was the expensive trace element, vanadium. The antidote is obviously unnecessary if stainless steel is not used for cooking, however convenient and long lasting it may be. Far better to use the older established and proven harmless pots and pans such as enamelled ware than risk health and life for the dubious benefits of longer life for the utensils and the risk of death from coronary thrombosis for oneself.

CHAPTER 19

DIAGNOSIS

Diagnosis is the art of discovering the presence of disease from the ability to correctly observe and interpret the signs and symptoms which are found by examination.

Two kinds of examination of the body can be undertaken for diagnostic purposes: they are—physical examination and chemical examination.

Physical Examination

The symptoms are elicited from the patient and compared with those learned as occurring in classical examples of disease. In this way a general term can be placed on the condition of the patient. The signs are observed in the patient at first hand by carrying out a thorough and methodical examination by means of : (*a*) Inspection, (*b*) Palpation, (*c*) Percussion, (*d*) Ausculation, and (*e*) Mensuration.

INSPECTION—this is done by examination of the parts by sight.

PALPATION—examination by feeling, using the fingers with varying pressure to examine as far as possible the different layers of tissue. A great deal of practice and experience will alone give efficiency in this.

PERCUSSION—this means striking or tapping and is done by placing the fingers of one hand on the part to be examined and tapping by a finger of the other hand.

AUSCULATION—this is using the ears in the detection of abnormality in the body. It can be done by placing the ear directly over the part of the body to be examined or by using a stethoscope.

MENSURATION—this is done by measuring the different parts of the body, e.g., muscles, and comparing with either the other normal side of your patient or if this is not possible, with what would generally be considered normal.

Carrying Out Physical Diagnosis

To properly carry out physical diagnosis, the part to be examined should be bare, and if a thorough examination is required, the patient should strip and lie on an examination table. The patient should of course be covered with a sheet and uncovered then as required. Care should be taken not to expose more of the body than is necessary, particularly when dealing with the opposite sex, and thus avoid embarrassment.

PALPATION will enable the practitioner to determine size, shape, consistency and mobility of parts. The muscles should be relaxed as far as possible, and abnormal tenderness or loss of feeling observed. Use pressure from the palmer surfaces of the fingers, gradually increasing or decreasing as required and watching the patient for signs of pain or distress.

PERCUSSION is best carried out by placing the second finger of the left hand in contact with the skin over the part to be examined. Strike the middle phalange of this finger with the tip of the second finger of the right hand, using firm, regular blows. Listen to the tone of the sound produced, i.e., pitch and intensity. Different sounds will be noted for different tissues of the body, and thus the examiner with experience can detect and diagnose abnormalities. A stethoscope can often be used to advantage. The bell of the stethoscope is placed between the little and fourth fingers of the left hand, holding it firmly against the skin while the percussion is done.

Sound examples:

Abdomen—a drum-like sound, long low pitched and fairly loud under normal conditions.

Lungs—More vibrating and of medium pitch.

Liver—Soft, short and high-pitched.

With this method different organs can be outlined on the

body with a grease pencil. This is auscultatory percussion and it is a good plan to practise this as often as possible on as many different people as possible.

AUSCULATION involves the use of the stethoscope which is designed mainly for examination of the heart and lungs. The sounds as magnified, enabling the examiner to easily determine varying conditions. The instrument should be held firmly on the chest, and held quite still during the examination as any movement will be magnified and sound in the instrument. A sound heart will produce a strong, regular beat which is heard when the instrument is placed over the apex. You will hear the systole and diastole of the heart, which are the characteristics related to the contracture of the organ and the closure of its valves.

The first sound of the heart is brought about by the ventricular systole and the closing of the tricuspid and mitral valves. This is a long, low-pitched sound. The second is at the beginning of the ventricular diastole, caused by the closing of the semi-lunar valves. This is a short, sharp sound. Together they form a sort of "Rub-dub". These two sounds are normally close together.

All variations in the quality of the heart muscles or in the action of the heart valves will result in a variation from normal in the sounds produced. A weak muscle, for example, will produce a weak first sound, and faulty closing of the valves will produce a blurred, rushing sound or slight wheezing known as a "murmur". From this can be diagnosed a leakage or regurgitation. If the sound is muffled it can signify an increase of pericardial fluid. If there is a first short, double sound like a gallop it will be indicative of cardiac weakness. When the flow of blood is obstructed by a faulty valve, this is termed "stenosis". Stenosis and regurgitation will produce enlargement of the heart with thickened walls which is known as "hypertrophy". If the heart, on the other hand, is overworked beyond its powers, it will cause dilation. In this case the heart enlarges with thin walls.

If the rest period of the heart becomes shortened, there is degeneration present. To complete the diagnosis of the heart, ask the patient to jump up and down a few times and then listen again. If there is faintness or cyanosis (blueness of the skin due to cardiac malfunction) the heart is inefficient.

The Lungs

During examination the patient should breathe deeply and evenly and as silently as possible. Use percussion and if there is decreased resonance, some consolidation will have taken place. If the sound is very dull, it will be indicative of fluid in the pleura or edema. Restricted respiratory movements may be due to rib adhesions or to subluxations or to pleural effusions, etc. Using the stethoscope, it will be found that normally expiration is louder and longer with a higher pitch than the sounds observed during inhalation. The instrument should be placed over the trachea of the large bronchi for this effect and if placed over the body of the lungs other than the right apex, the sounds will be reversed. Exaggerated sounds will indicate bronchial obstruction, atrophy or restricted activity of the lungs. If the air channels are obstructed for any reason, this will produce a whistling or snoring noise.

General Physical Examination

Having given detailed reminders of what to look for in the examination of the heart and lungs, some more general observations of what to look for in an overall physical diagnosis are now given:

1. Note the general appearance of the patient, observe posture, standing and sitting positions, rate of movement, mental condition and general behaviour regarding mannerisms, etc.
2. Examine the tongue for coating, etc., and note the colour, if any.
3. Study the face, expression, colour, etc., state of nutrition, eye colour and condition, etc.
4. Find out variations of temperature; if subject to night sweats, etc.

5. The rate, volume and regularity of the pulse should be noted—average rate is about 72 per minute. It is more rapid in women than men. Two or three fingers placed along the course of the radial artery with slight pressure are used for this purpose and take the rate over a full minute.

6. Carefully watch the respiratory movements in the chest and abdominal walls, observing depth and freedom as well as rate.

7. Examine the skin in detail and note moisture, surface, condition, presence of rashes, etc.

8. Examine and palpate the abdominal region, observing size and sensitivity, etc. You should only be able to feel the psoas muscles (insertion in the lesser trochanter of the femur), the lumbar vertebrae and abdominal aorta.

9. Examine and observe the movement of the apex of the heart, the strength, force and regularity, etc.

10. Examine the spinal column for defects, deformities, curvatures and all small deviations from normal.

11. If thought advisable, take the blood pressure of the patient. An instrument known as a sphygnomanometer or "manometer" is used for this purpose. They can be bought from surgical suppliers. Full instructions as to how to use these are usually presented with the instrument when purchased.

Indications of Signs Observed in the Examination

High temperature may indicate fever, infection, inflammation, toxaemia or nervous disturbances, tuberculosis, etc.

Loss of weight may be caused by insomnia, malnutrition, faulty metabolism, infections, etc.

The skin—in heart and lung disease the skin takes on a bluish colour. It is very pale in anaemia and in tuberculosis there is an artificial pink transparent colour of the cheeks. It is pale in arteriosclerosis. It is yellow in jaundice and toxaemia. It can have brown spots in chronic fevers and liver disorders. It has a peculiar odour in syphilis, cancer, Addison's disease and malaria. It will erupt in cases of toxaemia due to suppressive drug treatments and in acute infections as well as in some fevers, smallpox, etc. It will become inflamed and tender in acute rheumatic conditions or other inflammatory disturbances such as sprains, and will be hot, red and dry.

The Vertebrae

From abnormalities of the vertebrae or certain spinal groups may be diagnosed diseased conditions of various parts of the body which can be checked by further local investigation and examination. The following is a list of the vertebrae with parts of the body affected by them :

Organs and Parts	Spinal Nerve Centres
Head	1st to 6th cervical
Heart	3rd cervical to 5th dorsal
Intestines	9th dorsal to 5th lumbar
Kidneys	11th dorsal to 5th lumbar
Legs	12th dorsal to 5th sacral
Liver	6th to 12th dorsal
Lungs	1st to 9th dorsal
Larynx	1st and 2nd cervical
Pancreas	9th and 10th dorsal
Phrenic Nerve	2nd to 5th cervical
Peritoneum	1st and 2nd lumbar
Prostate Gland in males	10th dorsal to 5th lumbar
Spleen	9th and 10th dorsal
Trachea	5th and 6th dorsal

The above is not meant to be in any way an exhaustive survey but will give the reader a general idea since the whole theory of whether or not disease or disturbance of organs or parts can actually be produced by subluxations or deformities of the vertebrae, is open to question. Conversely, whether disease of an organ or part can produce deformity or slight deviation in the vertebrae, is also debatable. It is mentioned here because it is put forward as one of the theories of Osteopathy which claims to cure disease by manipulation of the vertebrae as outlined above. It is also true to say that many present-day Osteopaths do not accept this theory and they only claim to treat actual abnormalities with a view to restoring and maintaining mobility of joints and structures where these are normally mobile. It would take too long and it is not the function of this book to enter into any argument as to the viability of the theories connected with Osteopathy, which have in fact been going on since this form of physical treatment was first invented by Andrew Still in about 1864. One thing is certain, no harm can be done by giving good massage and soft tissue manipulation to the body, and in a later chapter an explanation is given of the methods used in this form of physical treatment. Osteopathy is a specialized therapy involving joint manipulation which can only be taught by regular attendance at a good school of Osteopathy and as such is quite outside the scope of this book.

Also outside the scope of this book is the teaching of the basic sciences of anatomy and physiology but this is not to say that a good knowledge of these subjects is not an essential for any would-be exponent of Naturopathic Practice. There are a great number of good text books on these subjects from simple guides to profound studies and the reader is certainly recommended to make a thorough study of them, if only as an advancement in self-knowledge.

Taking the Body Temperature

Finally, as far as physical diagnosis is concerned—the temperature of the patient should be taken. For this is required a clinical thermometer which most chemists sell. The usual way is to place the thermometer under the tongue for three minutes or so with the lips closed. It can also be placed under the armpit (the axilla) but this does not give a satisfactory reading. The best results are obtained by placing the thermometer in the anus. The temperature of a normally healthy man is about 98.4 but this can vary slightly in conditions of ordinary health.

If the temperature is below normal or sub-normal, say about 95° then a very serious condition is involved and anything from

93° down is almost certainly fatal. These sub-normal temperatures are usually found in cases of wasting diseases, diseases of the brain and spinal cord and in haemorrhages. Abnormally high temperatures signify fevers, etc., and 106° or more is liable to prove fatal.

Chemical Analysis

It is not possible to carry out the more difficult chemical examinations which involve the use of costly apparatus and laboratory conditions, in the ordinary consulting room or clinic. This equipment is beyond the scope or skill of the average person. However, the more usual chemical analysis of the urine can be done in most homes or consulting rooms, so we will explain these :

Urinalysis—if possible a 24 hour specimen should be obtained, otherwise one taken about midday. A drop of formalin added at the time of excretion will preserve the urine and prevent chemical changes after urination.

Urine tests for sugar are so widely known that it is not intended to deal with them here. Full instructions with the materials for these tests can be obtained from every chemist at a small cost and most diabetics for example, can easily make their own regular tests for sugar.

The presence of albumin is readily seen by bringing a small quantity of urine to the boil in a test tube over a bunsen burner. If albumin is present, there will be coagulation like the white of an egg. Another chemical test can be made by allowing a few drops of urine to trickle slowly down a test tube in which there are a few drops of nitric acid. If albumin is present, a white line will be precipitated where the urine and acid meet.

In a healthy individual, the colour of urine is clear and transparent, of a light amber colour. This does vary, of course, to some extent from one individual to another.

Usually the heavy meat eater will display a darker coloured urine than the vegetarian. A green colour indicates the presence of bile and points to a jaundiced condition, while dark brown indicates uric acid and rheumatic symptoms. Red means the presence of blood—can mean ulceration, bladder tumour, etc.

The average adult passes about three pints of urine in twenty-four hours and secretion is slowed down and almost halted during the hours of sleeping. The specific gravity is between 1011 and 1025 and increases in some cases of nephritis or with absorption of saccharine in the case of diabetes and in febrile conditions. It is decreased in kidney diseases and many nervous disorders. A litmus test should reveal a slight acidity although if the test is taken immediately after meals, an alkaline reaction will result.

Urea, chlorides and phosphates can also be found in the urine, and small quantities of indican and albumin, also uric acid and minute amounts of acetone.

Prognosis

From the foregoing it should be possible to work out a prognosis for the patient. This is a forecast of the duration and general course the disease will follow. The accuracy of this will naturally depend on the accuracy with which details of the patient's history, diagnosis, etc., have been taken. The good practitioner can usually make a very good prognosis and this communicated to the patient in advance and proved with the passing time and the achievement of cure, where this is possible, will serve to increase the faith and confidence of the patient in the practitioner, thus paving the way for a greater understanding between the two.

PART 5

PHYSIOTHERAPY

CHAPTER 20

MASSAGE

No treatise of Naturopathic Practice would be complete without the inclusion of massage as at least an auxiliary treatment. It is widely used by most practising naturopaths and is so beneficial even for the apparently healthy that no apology is made for giving details and instructions for its use here despite the fact that there are a few cases when it could in fact be contra-indicated.

Massage is given in many ways and for widely different purposes. The better known and more widely used techniques are described here. Broadly speaking, massage is composed of a number of different movements designed to have various effects on the body. It has been employed throughout the ages as a healing art and was brought to Greece from ancient Egypt. The Orientals were highly skilled operators many centuries before Christ.

Some movements are stimulating whilst others are relaxing in their effect and the choice of movement will be made with a view to securing the desired effect. For example, the highly strung type will need soothing and relaxing treatment while the flabby and indolent individual will need vigorous, stimulating techniques. Careful muscle treatment will retone the tissues and help in the expulsion of accumulated toxins in the exhausted athlete.

The whole art of massage depends upon the steady rhythm and pressure applied by the operator, and no massage can be remotely successful unless these two fundamentals are observed. Just as we all breathe with a steady rhythm and the heart beats with its own rhythm, so must the massage treatment be performed with a steady, even rhythm and consistent pressure as required in the individual case. Speed is not the object of good massage and this leads to jerky movements which are not conducive to good treatment.

Massage properly performed will promote the supply of blood to areas treated and assist in venous drainage which means a speeding up of used blood back to the heart and its re-oxygenation before setting out again to supply adequate nutrition to tissues of all kinds. In this way it assists in the expulsion of toxin of all kinds from tired muscle and brings a supply of fresh nutrients for their use. Fresh blood will be brought quickly to the surface of the skin which, being an organ of elimination, will also commence to play its part in this regenerative process. Massage to the extremities is particularly important as it is here that the blood supply becomes most sluggish and this is more especially true in older people and in the bedridden, infirm and aged. Too much attention cannot be paid to this and if all elderly folk whose movements become restricted through disability were given this treatment in a proper manner, there would be far less loss of limbs in the aged and they would remain much more active and less likely to become liabilities on society in general.

It is necessary to stress the importance of the use of the hands in good massage and avoiding as far as possible the various mechanical aids now so widely employed in this therapy. These are the lazy physiotherapist's "gimmicks". Nothing has yet been invented which will take the place of human hands. Throughout history it has been known that something more than warmth is generated by good massage when this is done by an operator who has the ability to convey confidence and optimism to his patient. No one has ever been able to define this something which may ultimately be found in the realms of metaphysics.

The treatment room should be pleasant and warm with a cheerful atmosphere. The antiseptic atmosphere and stark chromium-plated décor of the hospital is to be avoided. The plinth or couch should be about 2 ft. 6 in. high according to the operator's height, so as to prevent too much bending. It should be covered with a warm blanket and a fresh sheet supplied for each patient. The patient should remove all clothing as any type of restrictive clothing will impede the blood supply and completely defeat the objects of the treatment. Naturally, the patient will be properly covered with warm turkish towelling and only the areas being treated are exposed, the rest of the body being kept warm and relaxed.

Massage is of greatest benefit in cases of stiffness, sore muscles, numbness, paralysis, rheumatism, strains, sprains, etc., and it can be used to increase peristaltic action of the bowels to overcome constipation. The main object of massage is to restore and maintain function and mobility. The intelligent use of it can only result in benefit to many and various conditions, for through its medium it is possible to influence directly or indirectly every structure of the human body.

The Movements of Massage

There are five fundamental movements of massage, varied and adopted for use on various parts of the body :

    1. Effleurage (Stroking)
    2. Frictions (Rubbing)
    3. Petrissage (Kneading)
    4. Tapotement (Percussion)
    5. Vibrations (Shaking and trembling)

EFFLEURAGE is given by gliding the hand with long and even strokes over the muscle or group of muscles or tissues being treated. There are two modes of application—superficial and deep.

The light stroking movement aims only at a reflex effect. It should combine slowness with perfect rhythm and as little pressure as possible. It can be given in the centrapetal or centrifugal direction, that is in the direction of venous return or against it. It acts on the sympathetic nervous system and has a remarkably soothing effect.

Effleurage proper is only carried out in the centripetal direction or direction of venous return. It is performed with firm deep pressure and again perfect rhythm. It restores tone to the vasomotor system.

FRICTIONS—are carried out by using the palmer surfaces of the fingers or the thumbs. They are pressed firmly on the part and the movements are rapid and circular, keeping the fingers as springy as possible all the time. The joints, spine and abdomen benefit from this type of massage. It is of great value to the nerves, and it achieves absorption of local effusions, the stretching of adhesions, and breaking down of inflammatory conditions, etc.

PETRISSAGE—is a kneading, pressing, rolling and squeezing movement. It can be performed with one or two hands according to the type of petrissage being employed and the area to be treated. The general idea is to grasp the muscle or group of muscles and wring them out, holding them firmly and then releasing them. In this way blood waste, etc., is expelled from the area under treatment and on releasing, a new supply of fresh blood is admitted with fresh nutrition.

This is stimulating to the nervous system, blood vessels and glands and promotes cell exchange. It increases the supply of arterial blood.

TAPOTEMENT—is the rapid striking of the body with the hands or fingers. The blows are always given from the wrist and are short and quick. It is the most difficult group of movements to do successfully and there are four different kinds:

1. Hacking or chopping (for this the ulnar borders of the hands are used). This is done by each hand in rapid succession as are all these movements from the wrist so as to ensure that immediately the hand reaches the surface

being treated it is the end of the blow and no pain is caused the patient. These movements with the exception of tipping and tapping are never done over bony surfaces, but are used mainly over the larger muscle groups such as the hamstrings and the buttocks.

2. Tapping and Tipping or punctuation. This is done with the tips of the fingers and is of most use along the spine and on the sternum (breast bone).

3. Clapping and Cupping—here the open hands are used cupped to form a hollow. This is most useful for the superficial nerves and vessels of the skin as well as over organs like the liver and kidneys, and where there is plenty of soft, fleshy tissue.

4. Beating or Pounding—the part is here struck with the ulnar surfaces of the closed fists, used mainly on the buttocks and the lower extremities and over the sciatic nerve. It should not be used in cases of paralysis of the flaccid variety and where muscular spasm or hypertonicity amounting to a state of abnormal contraction is present. Nor should it be given in cases of nervous exhaustion, or in heart and nerve cases. It is of most value where muscular tone is present but deficient.

VIBRATIONS—These are given by placing the hand or fingers over the part and rapidly shaking by trembling movements with some degree of pressure. The position can be slightly modified round the area every minute or so. This type of treatment will increase the contractile power of muscles and is of great value in neuritis and neuralgia after the acute inflammatory stage is over. It is wonderful treatment for stimulating the circulation, glandular activity and the nervous plexuses. It is also very useful for constipation and it acts by increasing the peristatic action of the intestines. Take five or ten minutes for best results on the abdomen.

In carrying out massage, always treat muscles or groups of muscles and never whole limbs or parts at one time. For example, never massage the whole of the back at once but commence with the neck muscles and then work over the various groups of muscles in the back separately down to the lumbar region. After this the muscles which hold the spine in position, the *spinalis erectus muscles,* should be done. These will be found on either side of the vertebral column.

It is usual when carrying out a massage of the whole body to commence with the patient in the supine position and work on the toes first (good digital frictions and passive movements to put each joint through its complete range of movement). After this the foot with the metatarsal bones, then the ankle followed by mainly the muscle at the side of the shin (tibia) bone known as the *tibialis anitcus.* The knee joint is then carefully treated securing free movement of the kneecap (the patella). The thigh muscles are large muscles which require treatment with all the main massage movements outlined, while such areas as the foot will best be dealt with by effleurage and digital friction movements. The arm is then treated in the same way as the leg—all the muscle groups and joints separately, after which the chest with the pectoral muscles, the intercostal muscles, etc., followed by the abdomen with particular attention to this in cases of constipation. The patient is then turned over to the prone or face down position and the treatment again commenced from the foot to the top of the thigh, followed by the neck, and back, as outlined and the buttocks are treated last.

Contra Indications

To close this brief survey on massage treatment, there are listed here some of the conditions where it would be very unwise to carry out any kinds of massage and where in fact it is most definitely contra-indicated. These are mainly :

Skin affections, burns, sores, tumours and purulent inflammation, fevers, serious diseases of the circulatory system and blood diseases. Acute inflammatory conditions of the joints, pregnancy, menstruation (massage can be useful in cases of scant or retarded flow), acute bone diseases and of course in all conditions where there may be danger of producing haemorrhage.

Simple massage with a view to increasing circulation and metabolism can always be undertaken with confidence, but the treatment of deformities and serious lesions are properly the province of the properly trained osteopath or manipulative therapist. A great deal of harm can be done by unskilled manipulation of this kind, and anyone without the proper training would be ill advised to experiment with any manipulative techniques even though they may have been studied from a good text book. Osteopathic manipulative technique, as has already been stated, can only be taught in a practical way, by competent operators.

CHAPTER 21

MEDICAL ELECTRICITY

The complement of massage in Naturopathic Practice is Electrotherapy or Medical Electricity, and no study of massage would be complete without reference to the various ways in which electricity can be used to assist with physical treatments. It is essentially a part of physiotherapy and the details given here are intended to complete and round off theoretical background of Naturopathic knowledge. But as stated in the previous chapter, never allow the use of electrical "gimmicks" to take the place of good, honest massage. Electricity has a useful place as a part of physiotherapy but it is no substitute for a pair of hands properly employed.

Electricity

Electricity for our purpose may be described as a substance composed of rapidly moving electrons which will travel at the same speed as light, i.e. at 186,000 miles per second. This, of course, brings it into the realm of physics, governed largely by the relativity theory.

An electron is a fundamental of all matter pervading the entire cosmos, and every substance of which we so far have cognizance is composed of countless electrons grouped together in varying ways. In fact, one substance differs from another more or less on account of its varying rate of vibration.

Until the last century, it was believed that the atom was the smallest particle of indivisible matter, but we now know that even the atom is again subdivided into countless electrons. The electrons compose the substance of the atom. The negative electron has nearly ten times the velocity of the positive electron.

Insulators

Substances in which the nuclei are closest together are the best insulators as they possess an alignment of atoms which make it very difficult for the moving electrons to pass and they are deflected. These electrons always travel in straight lines until they collide with a positive nucleus when they are deflected, and travel again in a different direction. A great deal of heat is generated by the separation of the positive from the negative electrons in the atom. When a large number of negative electrons are taken from an atom, the potential is lowered, while the potential of the atom to which they escape is at once increased. This escape of electrons is known as an electrical charge, which results in a flow of electrical current.

Electricity is everywhere—in the air, in the earth, in all vegetation and in fact in every form of life and everything that we can think of which has some form of organized existence. In fact, it is a basic constituent of and a link between all four of the cardinal elements mentioned in an earlier part of this book. Electrical energy can be transposed into mechanical energy, into heat, light and sound but it can never be lost. It is the constant unchanging bridge which holds the four cardinal elements bound forever in relation to each other, each with this lowest common denominator.

We assume that the reader will have studied something of the basic laws of electricity and magnetism at school or college, and it is merely intended to refresh the memory here with some of the terms and definitions which are in use :

VOLT—is the unit of electro-motive force. It is the pressure exerted to force 1 ampere of current through a resistance of 1 ohm.

AMPERE—is the unit of electrical current. The strength or rate of flow is known as the amperage.

OHM—is the unit of electrical resistance. Some substances offer more resistance than others, and the best of these are known as good insulators while at the other end of the scale we have good conductors. The best insulator is air, followed by glass.

WATT—is the unit of electrical power. It is the amount of power produced by a current of 1 ampere under a force of 1 volt. Amperes multiplied by volts will provide the wattage.

When wires are used for return and lead conductors, this is known as a letallic circuit, and when the earth is used for the return current, it is known as a Ground Circuit or Earth Return.

Most people already know something of the value of electricity in the treatment of disease, and of how valuable it can be in assisting physiotherapists in a variety of ways. Life itself would seem to be a vibratory force, and when there is harmonious vibration of all the body cells, we are in a state of health. Disease is the result of discordant vibrations, and below a certain vibratory rate the body will die and begin to disintegrate, resolving itself once more to the fundamentals from which it came.

Treatments

When treatments are given to nerve centres, they are known as indirect treatments, and when applied directly to some organ or affected part, they are called Direct Treatments.

Electricity by means of various agents invented by man is able to help in the treatment of a variety of diseases, and with various instruments we are able to produce different kinds of currents, using them, as a result of experience, in the most suitable and advantageous ways.

GALVANISM is a continuous current set up by a machine usually used at low voltage (about 40) and of medium current value or even low current value. Here there are two contact points known as the positive and negative poles. Each pole produces active properties which are opposites :

Negative Pole—this attracts hydrogen, accumulates alkalines, dilates the arterioles and softens and liquifies tissues. It increases bleeding and is stimulating in effect.

Positive Pole—this attracts oxygen, contracts the arterioles and accumulates acids. It stops bleeding, hardens tissues and is sedative in its action.

Galvanic current generally stimulates metabolism and goes on acting for several days after the treatment. It is a good way of strengthening muscles by making use of a "make and break" system in the circuit. In this way, by the use of the positive pole, the muscle can be made to contract and expand rhythmically and so exercise and strengthen its tissues. When utilizing this current always make sure to use the correct electrode in the proper position. Treatment can be given to the various segments of the spine to influence the various organs and parts of the body which they affect as outlined previously. The electrodes take the form of pads for this purpose and can also be used to obtain spinal reflexes. This type of current is easily generated by dry cell batteries and can easily be moved about and used even in places where mains electricity is not available.

Static Electricity

This is produced by a revolving disc which most readers will remember from school days in the laboraory. It is pulsating current of very high voltage and very low amperage. This will also produce muscle contraction. The blood pressure is raised by this treatment, which also accelerates metabolism.

High Frequency

This is a very rapidly oscillating current of high voltage and low current value. The alternations are so rapid that the sensory nerves do not respond and it is very safe to use. It is produced by a leyden jar or other type of condenser. The strength of the current is measured by the length of the spark produced between the electrode and the skin. With these machines there are a variety of electrodes for different purposes. The electrode is kept in contact with the skin and moved about to prevent sticking. The average length of treatment is between ten and twenty minutes and details of a great many treatments are given with each machine. They can be bought at a reasonable price and are very portable for operation, using the usual mains supply.

When a spark is required, the tube may be passed over a sheet which is placed over the part to be treated. The length of the spark will then be the thickness of the material. The effect of this type of treatment is to increase the volume of blood and lymph to the parts, which will consequently improve nutrition to the areas. This is a form of cellular massage and acts on the nerves, tissues and cells. Make sure and keep the electrodes clean with a good germicide. The part so treated is also bathed in ozone which is highly beneficial. There is also a tube electrode specially used for generating ozone which can then be inhaled by the bronchial types and asthmatics, emphysemics and other respiratory sufferers. Fulguration can also be used with these machines and a special fulgurator electrode is supplied. It is held a space apart from the spot on which it is designed to direct the spark so as to produce the longest spark possible. This treatment is used for the removal of warts and other skin blemishes.

Diathermy

This is a high frequency current for producing heat in any part of the body and at any depth. It should never be used by the inexperienced as it can cause great harm where there is acute inflammation. It is, however, an excellent treatment for neuritis, neuralgia, lumbago, sciatica, arthritis, rheumatism and pneumonia, etc. It is applied by two pads which form the electrodes.

Sinusoidal

This is a smoothly alternating current of low voltage and high amperage. With a good apparatus it will give slow, rapid and surging sinusoidal currents. These are very much superior in effect to those produced by the faradic coil. It should never be used in cases of high blood pressure. It is of especial value where muscle stimulation is required and when both electrodes are used on the abdomen in cases of constipation due to motor insufficiency, the results will be splendid.

One great value of this treatment is that it will produce muscular contraction without the electrode having to be placed over the motor impulse. Usually one electrode is placed over the affected area and the other over the related spinal segment. This type of current is also used for electric baths.

Ultra Violet Rays

These rays are present in the light of the sun. They are among the shortest of the light waves and are called actinic or chemical and are the principal therapeutic rays of light. They bring about increased metabolism and exert a chemical action on the skin as distinct from the physical action produced by the heat rays. As was mentioned in the chapters on nutrition, they enable the body to manufacture its own calciferol or vitamin "D". These actinic rays act on the ergosterol present in the tissues of the skin and turn it directly into calciferol. Large doses should never be given at one time and frequent short doses are the best way of using these rays. They will be found very useful in the treatment of acne and psoriasis as well as other skin diseases. The first treatment should be of only about thirty seconds duration and gradually extended as toleration is increased to a maximum of ten to fifteen minutes. At all times both the patient and the operator should wear correct eye protection. Accurate exposures with regard to distance from the source of the rays can only be obtained from the manufacturers' guide as there are many types of ultra violet lamps on the market today, all having different grades of power. The old method of producing ultra violet rays by means of carbon electrodes is obsolete as far as medical use is concerned, although some of this type are still on sale for home use. The main drawback to these is that the smoke produced in making the ultra violet arc with carbon electrodes absorbs a great many of the valuable rays. Mercury vapour contained in quartz lamps is the usual equipment of this kind seen in clinics.

Radiant Heat

Probably the most useful and widely used product of electricity in so far as treatments are concerned. It can be used in many ways.

Even by keeping a patient in a room which is electrically heated to maintain room temperature, we are making use of radiant heat therapeutically. More specifically, we can apply heat of this kind to the patient directly and apply it externally to any part of the body. It can be concentrated on particular muscles or regions where heat treatment is required and in our chapter on Hydrotherapy where the use of hot water bottles was advocated outside a cold pack, this was making use of radiant heat.

It is especially useful in dispelling inflammations in rheumatism, sciatica, etc., by producing relaxation of muscles and tissues, and is of great benefit immediately prior to massage. It can be prescribed over long periods. It is very safe to use.

Infra Red

These are much longer heat rays than radiant heat and are more deeply penetrating as the skin offers less resistance to them owing to their reaching the surface in parallel lines. They are used in the same way as is radiant heat and for the same purposes, also being very safe in use.

Ultra Sonic

This is another form of electrical treatment for inducing heat at depth. It has many advantages in use and is another very safe way of treatment. The sound heads can also be used for electrical water treatments and it has proved beneficial in all the rheumatic cases. There is always a good instruction book supplied with ultra sonic apparatus but it is quite expensive to buy.

Chromotherapy

In some ways this is the Cinderella of electrical treatments and is not given the use it deserves. Of course, there is still a great deal of research to be done as to the effects of various colour rays on the human organism and how they differ when used exclusively, one from the other. Some authorities say that there is no physiological effect and that the results are purely psychological. This, however, should not prevent their use as even though the results may be only psychological, if they are good then obviously chromotherapy is good treatment and it is a well-known fact that a good percentage of disease in human beings is of psycho-somatic origin.

Practical treatment consists mainly in confining the patient to rooms in which only one colour or a special blend of primary colours is present, or in treating parts of the body directly by concentrating beams of specific colour or colours on them.

A guide as to the general effects and indications produced, as far as they have been confirmed to date, is as follows:

GREEN—this is soothing to nerves generally and good for all those who suffer from hypertension.

RED—this is stimulating to the nerves and blood. It is useful in anaemia, paralysis, tuberculosis and various kinds of debility.

REDDISH ORANGE—is useful in cancerous and malignant growths. Good too for the skin and will help to clear up some forms of skin disease and certain types of eruptions.

YELLOWISH ORANGE—is stimulating, as are yellow and orange used alone. They have been found beneficial in digestive disorders, constipation and female pelvic disorders.

PILLAR BOX RED—has been found of great value in impotency in the male and has a generally stimulating effect on the male sex organs.

PASTEL BLUE—has been of great help in cases of bad memory and it has been found that concentrated study and other mental faculties are encouraged by this colour.

CHAPTER 22

CONCLUSION

Final Notes and Advice

This book has been written in an effort to present a complete working knowledge of naturopathy. It has not, like so many, merely given a list of various diseases with accounts of treatments for each, which often seem to appear so similar as to be almost identical, so that by reading the treatment for the first disease the treatment for each and every one that follows is known in advance. A thorough grasp of the principles here laid down should provide the reader with material from which a good specific treatment can be worked out along naturopathic lines and according to the long established principles of this type of healing. The reader should have a thorough knowledge of the application of food and its relation to health and be in a position to work out the best possible diet as part of a treatment for almost any type of disease. He will have a knowledge of physical medicine and also be in a position to use his own intelligence to the utmost in investigating any patient's condition, drawing conclusions as to the cause of any disease without having to rely on some outside opinion which may or may not be reliable.

The only real systems of natural healing which are not dealt with in any detail in this book are those of herbal medicine and homoeopathy with the biochemic tissue salts. These are long studies in themselves and would provide the material for further volumes. They have not been omitted because they are not important and the reader is strongly advised to gain for himself a knowledge of these therapies which are so often useful as natural healing agents.

However, even without a knowledge of either herbal medicine

or homoeopathy, a knowledge has been gained on which can be formulated sound constructive treatment so that where the possibility of cure exists, it can be obtained.

One last word—do not be content with reading. Put ideas into practice. Theory without methodology is useless. The Greeks achieved their unique place in the history of mankind by a training in, and the practical use of, their powers of observation. Train yourself to be observant at all times. Life is movement and nothing in this world of ours stands still.

Be always ready to add to your store of learning and be always ready to serve your fellow men. Observe any new fact which presents itself. You could be the first one in history to discover some little detail which could make all the difference between failure and success with even an established treatment of some well known disease. Remember also that the greatest fault of our present age is specialization. No man can ever know every-thing—this is true. We are finite but we can endeavour to hold in our minds as much as possible at all times.

We can, as we have been taught, train our senses to observe and collate as much information as possible about a patient. We can train our brains and minds to collate this information, which will instruct us exactly in the best treatments to employ in order to bring out a cure wherever possible in any given set of conditions.

A good all-round knowledge of the human animal and of the laws which govern his life on this planet will be found of far more value in treatment than a specialized knowledge of some specific aspect of disease or a wide knowledge of some particular aspect of the human body to the detriment of the rest.

Life is a totality and any patient is a totality. This should never be forgotten and neither should it be overlooked that every patient is a thinking individual, however imperfectly he may think. He needs to be taken into the confidence of the prac-titioner as well as being given confidence in himself. The known effects of any treatment should always be explained, and some idea given as to the results likely to be achieved, before it is embarked upon. The various aspects of a treatment should, for this reason, always be fully explained as they have been explained in this book. Never be afraid of disease. This is negative. Never think of disease. Think only of health and of how this can best be obtained.

There is one final therapy on which we have not touched in so many words, but one which may well make the difference between success and failure. This is INDUCED SUGGESTION and AUTO-SUGGESTION. Too little use is made of this wonderful method of healing and inducing confidence which was expounded by the famous Frenchman, Emil Coué. First of all, do your utmost to induce the idea that it is possible for your patient to get well. Go further than this, tell him to use a phrase such as "EVERY DAY IN EVERY WAY I GET BETTER AND BETTER".

This phrase should be repeated at least twenty times every night after going to bed and when the consciousness is dormant —in that state between sleeping and waking. If this is done you will be amazed at the wonderful results that can be achieved in a very short time even with the worst types of illness.

Induced suggestion can be given to the patient by having him lie on the examination table as relaxed as possible. The room should be warm and lit by a soft, subdued light (chromotherapy can play a part here). Gentle massage of the effleurage type can be employed on the spine while the suggestions required can be induced. A soft, well-modulated voice should be employed for this, and when the treatment is over, the patient should be given instructions for carrying out auto-suggestion himself at home.

Nothing now remains but to wish every reader success, whether it be in self-treatment or in the treatment of others—friends, relations or patients. Only the truly dedicated individual will succeed. The rewards are among the greatest that can be bestowed on any human being—those of seeing your fellow men suffer less and being educated to a healthier, saner, more constructive way of life.

GLOSSARY AND INDEX

GLOSSARY

ACTINIC. From the Greek "aktinos"—a ray—which we use in respect of those rays from the sun which have a chemical as distinct from a physical effect. The ultra-violet and shorter waves of the spectrum.

ALCHEMIST. Was principally a mediaeval chemist or doctor who in addition to seeking cures for various disease conditions was preoccupied in trying to find a method by which base metals such as lead could be transmuted to gold. He was also concerned in the search for Eternal Youth.

ALKALOIDS. Are extractive agents of various plants having a therapeutic action. Being natural nitrogenous organic bases they combine with acids to form crystalline salts. There are very few alkaloids to be had from animal sources; the best known being adrenalin.

ALTERATIVE. Is a herbal medicine which can correct a toxic condition of the blood without being a purgative or a laxative. A fast can have an alterative action on the blood.

AMINO-ACID. Is an organic acid derived by the digestive processes from proteins which the body can then use as nutrients for building into various tissues and organs.

ANTIBIOTIC. Anti-life. It is used generally to describe medicaments obtained from micro-organisms which are capable of destroying bacteria in the human body.

ARTERIOLE. A very small artery.

BACTERIOSTATIC. Is a substance which inhibits the growth by multiplication of bacteria.

BIOCHEMISTRY. Is the chemistry of living structures and the life processes and should not be confused with the biochemistry of Dr. Schüssler which in reality is a form of Homoeopathy and deals with only twelve tissue salts when in fact there are many more than this in the human body.

BRIGHT'S DISEASE. Discovered by Dr. Bright early last century and used to describe disease conditions of the kidney which cause the presence of albumin in the urine and dropsical symptoms. It is the same disease as nephritis.

CARCINOGENIC. Used to describe substances which can have cancer causing properties.

CORONARY THROMBOSIS. In cases of diseased coronary arteries the blood is considerably slowed up in its passage through the blood vessels and clots, cutting off the blood supply to the heart with often fatal results.

DECOCTION. This is a herbal preparation made by placing the fresh green or dried herb or plant in boiling water and simmering for a given length of time, allowing to cool and then straining off the liquor for use as a medicine.

DISSEMINATED SCLEROSIS. Is a disease which usually makes slow progress with symptoms which may not be noticeable for some time. It is caused by small patches of hard connective tissue forming in the brain and spinal cord. In the later stages of the disease forms of paralysis and tremors are produced.

ELECTRON. A particle far more minute than an atom and having a charge of electricity which is indisoluble from it.

ELEMENT. The basic essential of anything and we use the term to describe the basic substances of matter from which compounds are built, also it is used in reference to the Cardinal Elements of Air, Earth, Fire and Water from which the ancient alchemists supposed everything to be derived.

EMPHYSEMA. This is a disease of the lungs caused by abnormal distention of the air cells which break down and run together. It often follows as a sequel to chronic asthma or bronchitis.

ENZYME. A chemical ferment made by living cells, e.g. ptyalin in the saliva used in the digestive processes. They help to break down proteins into amino acids for use by the body in its rebuilding and repair processes.

FULGURATION. This is a lightning spark produced by High

Frequency treatment and used therapeutically for the removal of warts, etc. from the skin.

HERBAL INFUSION. A tea made with fresh or dried herbs or plants. Boiling water is poured over the herb—the quantity of each depending on the strength of the infusion required. On cooling the infusion is strained and taken as a medicine or it can be taken as a hot tea, etc.

HOMOEOPATHY. A system of medicine based on the law of similium (similia similius curantur). Drugs which in their crude state will produce symptoms in a healthy individual which are akin to the symptomology of the disease in a sick person are those which in a minute dose after trituration or attenuation will produce a stimulus to the Vital Force of the sick person in the direction of recovery. It was founded by Dr. Samuel Hahnemann in the late 1700's.

HORMONE. Or autocoid of a stimulating type is a substance which is absorbed into the blood (usually secretions of the endocrine glands) to affect tissues and organs in various parts of the body.

MIASM. A term used by Hahnemann to describe chronic or deep seated (rather than long lasting) taints in the blood which he classified into three basic categories—Psora, Psychosis and Syphilis.

MINERALS. These for our purpose mean the Elements which are found in the ash of food after combustion.

OSTEOPATH. A practitioner of Osteopathy which is a system of physical treatment in which diseases are treated by the manipulation of bone structures to correct maladjustments thus restoring the bodily functions and paving the way to health.

PARALYSIS AGITANS. Or shaking paralysis is a form of progressive muscular atrophy.

PARKINSON'S DISEASE. Is another name for paralysis agitans.

PEPTONE. Is a very simple compound of amino acids and takes the form of a whitish powder produced by the action of acids in digestion or artificially on meat or other proteins. It is soluble.

POLIOMYELITIS. Is an infectious disease caused by a virus which attacks the spinal cord and brain. Epidemics usually happen in the Autumn in this country.

POLYPEPTIDE. A group of amino acids less complex than peptones.

PROLAPSE. Usually used to describe a dropped condition of the womb or rectum.

PROTEOSES. Rather more complex substances than peptones described above.

PSYCHOSOMATIC. A term used to describe disease in which the physical symptoms are caused by mental disturbances.

SUBLUXATION. A partial dislocation and is a term used by Osteopaths in connection with deformities of the vertebrae.

SYNERGIST. A substance which has to be present in the body before bio-chemical combinations can take place to facilitate assimilation. The equivalent of catalysis.

TOXINS. Are poisonous substances which occur in the body either as a result of the presence of bacteria or the accumulation of wastes on which bacteria can thrive.

TRACE ELEMENTS. Are essential nutrients of the body although only required in very small amounts.

TUBERCLE BACCILUS. Or Mycobacterium Tuberculosis is the germ responsible for the disease of this name.

VEGAN. Is a person who in addition to being a vegetarian also abstains from all kinds of dairy produce.

VITAMINS. Are substances often complex which are required in minute quantities by the body. They are present in natural foods and if deficient either as a result of loss through the processing of food or for other reasons, can be the cause of various diseases.

VIRUS. Is the name given to the causative agent of diseases such as influenza, yellow fever, etc. It is small enough to pass through the pores of a colloidon filter.

INDEX

A

"A"vitamin, 60, 73, 74, 75, 109
Abnormalities, 156
Abscess, 42, 144
Accident, 24
Acetone, 159
Actinic, 172
Achromatin, 141
Adrenal Medulla, 85
Aeschylus, 38
Air, 47
Albumin, 158, 159
Alchemists, 47
Alkalis, 60
Alkaloids, 150
Alcohol, 28, 60, 150
Alcoholic drinks, 96
Alfalfa, 76
Allopathic disease classification, 22, 27
Allopathic medicine, 27, 32, 33, 43, 50
Alpha tocopheral, 75
Alterative, 87
Aluminium, 150
Amino acids, 57
Amoebae, 139
Amoeboid cell, 140
Amitosis, 141
Amperage, 168
Ampere, 168
Anabolism, 55, 56, 59
Anaemia, 64, 67, 81, 107, 144, 174
Anatomy, 21, 157
Analysis (chemical), 158
Aneurine hydrochloride, 77
Animal cells, 140
Androsterone, 85
Antibiotics, 110
Anti-neuritic, 77
Anti-rhacitic, 74
Anti-scorbutic, 81
Appendicitis, 28, 133

Appetite, 119
Apples, 66, 95, 106, 107
Apollo, 47
Apricots, 66, 95
Architects, 30, 48
Arsenic, 64
Art, 38, 48
Arterioles, 85
Arthritis, 81, 95
Asclepius, 48
Ascorbic acid, 80–82
Aspirin, 106
Asthma, 72, 74, 171
Assimilation, 36, 41, 49, 57
Athens, 30
Atrophy, 144, 154
Auscultatory percussion, 153
Average weight, 119, 120
Axilla, 157
Auto-suggestion, 177

B

"B₁" vitamin, 77, 78, 109
"B₂" vitamin, 77, 109
"B₆" vitamin, 78
"B₁₂" vitamin, 68
Back strain, 131
Bacteria, 32, 42, 59
Bacteriostatic, 81, 82
Balanced diet, 61
Balkans, 112
Bananas, 77, 95
Barium, 64
Baths, 88, 126, 127, 128, 129, 130
Béchamp, 32
Beet tops, 109
Beri beri, 77
Big drink day, 93, 101, 102
Bilberry, 106
Biochemistry, 31, 33, 79
Biochemists, 57
Biotin, 79
Birth, 49

Blackcurrants, 81, 97, 106
Bladder, 131
Blood, 41, 44, 48, 58, 60, 64, 163
Blood pressure, 125, 155, 170, 171
Body temperature, 157
Borage, 71
Brain, 77
Breathing, 48, 49
Bright's disease, 116
Brittle bones, 70
Bromine, 65
Bronchial obstruction, 154
Bronchitics, 137
Bronchii, 154
Bronchitis, 109, 137
Brussels sprouts, 66, 71
Buck wheat, 82
Building, 38
Burns, 74
Butter, 66
Buttermilk, 110, 112

C
"C" vitamin, 80, 81, 82
Cabbage, 98
Calciferol, 94, 172
Calcium, 62, 63, 65, 66, 74, 106
Calories, 116, 120
Cancer, 42, 68, 142, 145, 146, 174
Cane sugar, 58
Capillaries, 36, 60
Capillary fragility, 82
Carbohydrates, 55, 57, 58, 59, 60, 61, 77, 120
Carbon, 56, 61, 63, 84, 85
Carbon (Electrodes), 172
Carbonate salts, 63
Carcinogenic, 90
Cardinal elements, 47, 49
Cardiac malfunction, 154
Cardiovascular disease, 75
Carnivorous, 117
Carotene, 60, 73, 109
Carrots, 95, 109, 111
Casein, 56
Castor oil, 137
Cataract, 70
Catabolism, 55, 59
Catalysis, 59
Catarrhal, 128, 148
Cauliflower, 66, 71
Celery, 66, 98, 106, 107
Cells, 41, 140, 141, 142, 143
Cellulose, 59

Cell division, 141
Cell structure, 139
Cellular massage, 171
Cereals, 54, 77, 78
Cheese, 96
Chemical analysis, 158
Cherries, 107
Chickweed, 133
Chlorine, 62, 65, 66
Cholera, 112
Choline, 79
Chromium, 68, 150
Chromotherapy, 173, 174
Chromatic threads, 141
Chronic (Disease), 24, 25, 123
Cinchona, 34
Circulatory system, 36
Citrin, 82
Citric acid, 107
Civilizations, 30
Clinical, 157
Clothing, 148, 149
Coal tar, 106
Cobalt, 64, 68
Cocoa, 107
Cod, 116
Cod liver oil, 116
Coffee, 96
Colds, 43
Colitis, 135
Collagen, 81
Colon, 135
Colonic irrigation, 133, 134, 135, 136
Colour therapy, 173, 174
Comfrey, 71
Common cold, 81
Compresses, 106, 124, 132
Consciousness, 177
Condensation, 59
Congenital, 25, 143
Congestion, 128
Constipation, 112, 116, 133, 162, 174
Contagious, 143
Constitutional disease, 143
Constructive forces, 27
Convulsions, 129
Copper, 67, 68
Corn oil, 116
Coronary thrombosis, 146, 150
Corticosterone, 85
Cortex, 85
Cosmos, 29

Coué (Emil), 177
Cranberries, 107
Crisis (Healing), 26, 32, 44, 45
Crisis (Disease), 26
Culture, 38, 48
Cure, 43
Currants, 106
Cyanosis, 154
Cytoplasmic changes, 143
Cyst, 145

D

"D" vitamin, 73, 74, 75, 172
Dandelion, 66, 71
Dates, 95
Debility, 87, 174
Decoction, 124
Democratic, 30
Depleted vitality, 114
Dermatitis, 78
Diabetes, 115, 158, 159
Diagnosis, 51, 151–9
Diarrhoea, 78
Diastole, 153
Diathermy, 171
Diet, 49, 52, 53, 54, 82, 95, 97, 148
Diphtheria, 108
Disease, 19, 20, 24, 25, 26, 32, 33,
  53, 141, 143, 147
Disease crisis, 26
Disseminated Sclerosis, 68
Douches, 131
Dramatists, 30
Dropsy, 95
Dry day, 92, 93, 99, 100, 101
Ductless glands, 83

E

"E" vitamin, 75
Ear, 131
Earth return, 169
Eczema, 24, 123, 172, 174
Edema, 145, 154
Education, 38
Effleurage, 162, 163, 177
Eggs, 54, 78, 96, 98
Egg yolk, 77
Egypt, 30, 160
Elder flowers, 133
Electricity, 167
Electro-motive-force, 168
Electrons, 167, 168
Electrotherapy, 52, 167–74
Elements, 56, 57, 61, 62, 67, 72

Elixir, 84
Embolism, 145
Emmanuel Schroth, 93
Emphysemic, 171
Enamelled ware, 150
Endemic, 143
Endive, 98
Endocrine, 83
Endothelial, 141
Enema, 87, 88
Energy, 47
Enzymes, 59, 110
Epidemic, 143
Epsom salts, 128, 131, 136
Erythema, 78
Eskimo, 21
Etheric membrane, 29
Etiology, 147
Excesses, 52, 150

F

Failing sight, 70
Falling hair, 69
Fainting, 87
Faradic coil, 171
Fast, 86, 87, 88, 89
Fasting, 52, 55, 86, 91
Father Kneipp, 123, 124
Fats, 55, 58, 59, 60, 61, 120
Fatty degeneration, 145
Ferments, 59
Fevers, 42, 44, 132, 145
Fibrin, 56
Fibrositis, 95
Figs, 95
Filtrate factors, 62, 76
Finite, 29
Fire, 47
Fish, 96, 98, 116
Fish oils, 73
Flesh foods, 117
Flowers of sulphur, 137
Folk herbs, 124
Food classification, 55
Food reform, 53
Formalin, 158
Frictions, 162, 163
Fruits, 54
Fulguration, 171
Functional disease, 143

G

Gall bladder, 107
Gall stones, 107

Galvanism, 169, 170
Gangrene, 145
Garlic, 109
General debility, 87
Genito urinary (Disease), 129
Germs, 32, 33, 43
Giant cells, 140
Glands, 83
Globutin, 56
Glucose, 58, 59
Gluten, 56
Glycerine, 60, 137
God of Medicine, 47
Golden seal, 135, 137, 138
Gonads, 84
Gooseberries, 107
Grapefruit, 95, 107, 108
Grape cure, 105, 107
Grape wine, 97
Gravity douche, 87, 134
Greece, 30, 38, 113, 160
Greeks, 21, 30, 39, 56, 176
Green, 174
Ground circuit, 169
Growth, 49
Growth cells, 42

H
"H" vitamin, 79
Haemorrhage, 76, 146, 158
Haemorrhoids, 131
Haddock, 116
Hahnemann, 25, 31
Hair, 69
Halibut liver oil, 116
Harmony, 20, 39, 41
Heart disease, 123
Headaches, 44
Healing crisis, 44, 45
Health, 19, 20, 28, 49
Health Food Stores, 54
Heart beat, 48
Heat, 47, 48, 171, 173
Hemlock, 29
Herbal infusion, 133, 135, 138
Herbal medicine, 20, 31, 71, 175
Herbivorous, 117
Heracleitus, 38
Heredity, 42, 143
Hesperidin, 82
High frequency, 170
High temperature, 155
Hip joint, 133
Hippocrates, 30, 39

Homoeopathy, 20, 31, 147, 175, 176
Honey, 97, 109
Hormones, 83
Horsetail, 71
Hospital, 28, 37
Hound's tongue, 71
Housing, 148, 149
Hungarian pepper, 82
Hydrastis, 135, 137
Hydrocarbons, 60
Hydrogen, 56, 61, 81, 84, 85
Hydrolysis, 59
Hydrotherapy, 32, 49, 52, 88, 106, 108, 111, 122–38, 173
Hyoplasm, 140
Hyperaemia, 146
Hyperchromatic, 142
Hyperpiasia, 145
Hyperthyroidism, 85
Hypertrophy, 145, 153
Hyperchondriac, 19
Hypertension, 174
Hypochromatic, 142
"H" 3., 80

I
Ibis, 134
Ideology, 118
Immunity, 43
Impotence, 68, 107, 131, 174
Indican, 159
Indigestion, 78
Induced suggestion, 177
Infectious diseases, 73, 81, 143
Infinity, 29
Infantile death rate, 123
Inflammation, 42, 43, 146, 173
Infra red, 173
Inhibitions, 150
Infusion, 124
Injury, 24
Insanity, 42
Inositol, 79
Inspection, 151
Insulators, 168
Insulin, 84
Intensive breeding, 54
Interstitial, 144
Intestines, 59
Iodine, 65
Iron, 33, 62, 64, 66, 69, 81, 106
Ischaemia, 146

J
Joint manipulations, 157

K

"K" vitamin, 75, 76
Kale, 66
Karyokinesis, 141
Karyorrhexis, 143
Kelp, 136
Kidney disease, 128
Kidneys, 77, 85, 108, 128
Kinetic energy, 59

L

Lactic acid, 113
Lactoflavine, 77, 78
Large Bronchii, 154
Lassitude, 77, 87
Law of sevens, 34, 35
Laws of nature, 26
Leeks, 66
Lemons, 66, 95, 97, 106
Letallic circuit, 169
Lettuce, 66, 75, 98, 109
Leucocyte, 140
Leukaemia, 146
Life, 28, 36
Light, 47, 48, 49
Lime phosphate, 63
Lindlahr (Dr), 20, 34
Linoleac acid, 79
Litmus, 159
Liver, 73, 77, 107, 152
Local packs, 132
Longevity, 117
Loss of weight, 155
Lower back strain, 131
Lowered vitality, 78
Lumbago, 131
Lunatic, 48
Lungs, 77, 154, 156
Lungwort, 71
Lymph, 41, 44, 60, 63

M

Macrocosm, 47
Magnesium, 62, 63, 64, 66, 69
Magnesium phosphate, 64
Magnesium sulphate, 126
Maintenance cells, 142
Malic acid, 106, 107
Man, 47
Manganese, 68
Manometer, 155
Massage, 126, 160–66
Meat, 114, 115, 117, 118
Medical electricity, 167–74

Medicated baths, 127, 128
Medicine, 27, 38
Menstruation, 165
Mensuration, 151, 152
Mental depression, 103
Mental state, 149, 174
Menthol, 127
Metabolism, 55, 56, 64, 65, 69, 72, 75, 78, 79, 84, 87, 95, 110, 125, 170
Metaphysical, 162
Metaproteins, 57
Metchnikof, 112
Methodology, 20, 26, 176
Mercury vapour, 172
Miasms, 25, 42, 45, 123
Micro nutrients, 82, 84, 105
Microcosm, 47
Milk, 110–13
Milk products, 113
Mineral oils, 59
Minerals, 63, 72
Mint, 127
Mitosis, 141
Mitral Stenosis, 142, 153
Molasses, 137
Mono diets, 104, 105, 106, 110, 114
Moon, 48
Mud compresses, 136
Multipolar Mitrosis, 142
Muscles, 77, 78
Muscular Dystrophy, 78
Mushrooms, 96
Murmur (Heart), 153
Myosin, 56

N

Natural law, 24, 26
Naturopathic hydros, 123
Necrosis, 146
Nephritis, 159
Nerve cells, 77
Nerve centres, 156
Nervous exhaustion, 42
Nettles, 133
Neuritis, 128
Nicotinic acid, 78
Nitric acid, 158
Nitrogen, 56, 57, 61, 84, 85
Nose, 131
Nuclear network, 141
Nucleus, 140
Nuts, 95

O

Oak bark, 136

Oats, 77
Oestrin, 84
Ohm, 168
Oils, 59, 60
Oil soluble vitamins, 73, 74, 75, 76
Olive oil, 137
Olympic games, 39
Omnilateral, 19
Omniverous, 117
Onions, 109
Orange diet, 106, 107
Oranges, 81, 95, 107
Organic, Preface, 34, 144
Organs, 156
Osmotic pressure, 63
Osteoid arthritis, 81
Osteopathy, 20, 31, 49, 50, 106, 157
Ovaries, 84
Over-indulgence, 127
Overstrain, 128
Oxalic acid, 107
Oxydation, 77
Oxygen, 56, 60, 61, 63, 77, 84, 85, 170
Ozone, 171

P

"P" vitamin, 82
Palpation, 151, 152, 155
Pancreas, 60, 84
Pandemic, 144
Pantothenic acid, 79
Paprika, 82
Para-amino-benzoic-acid, 79, 80
Paralysis, 162, 174
Paralysis agitans, 78
Parathyroid, 85
Parkinson's disease, 78
Parsley, 66
Parsnips, 95
Pastel blue, 174
Pasteur, 32
Patella, 165
Pathological change, 139
Pathology, 21, 51, 52, 139–46
Peaches, 66, 95
Peanuts, 75
Pears, 95, 106, 107
Penicillin, 81
Pepper, 107
Peptones, 57
Percussion, 151, 152, 153, 154
Periodic (Disease), 144
Peristaltic action, 162, 163

Permeable, 140
Petrissage, 162
Phagocytes, 141
Philosophy, 20, 23, 40, 45, 48, 50, 51, 90, 96
Phosphoric acid, 66
Phosphorus, 56, 61, 62, 63, 64, 66, 69, 74, 84, 106
Physical action, 57
Physical examination, 151–7
Physical treatment, 157
Physiology, 21, 157
Physiotherapy, 31, 52, 108, 111, 160–6
Piles, 135
Pillar box red, 174
Pine bath, 137
Pineal body, 85
Pineapple, 108
Pituitary, 84
Plant cells, 140
Plant protein, Introduction
Plasma membrane, 140
Pleura, 154
Plums, 107
Poison, 24, 42, 66
Poliomyelitis, 90
Politics, 38
Polyhedral cells, 140
Polyneuritis, 77
Polypeptides, 57
Posture, 154
Potassium, 62, 63, 65, 66, 84, 90
Potassium sulphate, 137
Potatoes, 77, 95, 109
P.P. factor, 78
Pregnancy, 78
Prognosis, 51, 159
Prolapse, 131
Prostate gland, 136
Proteins, 36, 55, 56, 57, 58, 59, 61, 116, 118, 120
Proteoses, 57
Prothrombin, 76
Protoplasm, 56, 57, 140
Protruding eyes, 85
Prunes, 98, 107
Psoas muscle, 155
Psora, 42
Psoriasis, 74
Psychic, 24, 30, 35
Psychic activity, 48
Psychosomatic, 123, 174
Psychotherapy, 32, 174

Purgative enema, 137
Pulse, 155
Pyrodoxin, 78

Q

Quantitative diet, 119, 120
Quartz lamp, 172
Quinine, 34

R

Radiant heat, 172, 173
Raspberries, 106
Raw foods, 118
Rectum, 131
Red, 174
Red currants, 106
Reddish orange, 174
Regurgitation, 153
Rensoic acid, 107
Repressions, 150
Respirations, 77
Respiratory, 73, 74, 128
Restricted diet, 88, 89
Rheumatic disease, 68, 72, 95, 105,
    106, 136, 172, 173
Rheumatic joints, 133, 136
Rheumatism, 126, 162, 172, 173
Rhubarb, 107
Riboflavine, 77, 78
Rickets, 74
Rosehips, 81
Roughage, 59
Round cells, 140
Russia, 112
Russian bath, 127
Rutin, 82
Rhythm, 26, 34, 40, 48, 92, 161

S

Saccharine, 159
Salads, 98
Salicin, 106
Salt, 63, 131
Saponifiable, 60
Sauna, 127
Saw Palmetto, 136
Sciatica, 95, 131
Science, 38
Schroth Cure, 91, 52, 95, 99, 101,
    105
Schroth, Emmanuel, 93
Schroth, Johann, 91, 93
Schroth pack, 91, 131
Sculptors, 30, 48

Scurvy, 81
Sea salt, 131, 136
Seaweed, 131, 136
Self repair process, 20
Senile, 74
Senility, 37
Sensory nerves, 170
Sex gland, 83
Silica, 68, 69, 70, 71, 72
Silicon, 62, 64, 66, 67, 69
Sinusoidal, 171
Skin, 45, 78, 81, 155, 156
Skin eruptions, 128
Sleep, 148
Sleeping, 177
Small drink day, 92, 93, 101, 102
Soap, 60, 73, 129, 130
Socrates, 29, 37
Sodium, 62, 63, 65, 69, 106
Solar, 48
Sorrel, 107
Sound head, 173
Sour milk, 112, 113
Spas, 123
Spasms, 129
Specific, 144
Sphygmanometer, 155
Spinach, 109
Spinalis erectus muscles, 165
Spinal nerves, 156
Spine, 170
Spindle cells, 140
Spleen, 77, 85
Spongy gums, 81
Sporadic, 144
Sprains, 162
Straight nature cure, 31
Stainless steel, 150
Starch, 58, 59, 61
Static electricity, 170
Steam bath, 127
Stenosis, 153
Sterility, 75
Stethoscope, 151, 153
Stiffness, 162
Stomach, 131, 137, 138
Strains, 162
Strawberries, 66, 106
Strontium, 64
Subacute disease, 144
Subchronic disease, 144
Subluxations, 42, 156
Sugar metabolism, 84
Sulphur, 56, 61, 62, 64, 66, 84

Sunflower seed, 116
Suppressions, 150
Suppressive ointment, 123
Sweat pack, 132
Swollen feet, 133
Sycosis, 42
Symptomology, 146, 147
Symptoms, 51, 124, 147
Synergist, 34, 41, 64
Syphilis, 42
Systole, 153

T

Tapotement, 163, 164
Tartaric acid, 107
Tea, 96, 107
Tension, 128
Testis, 75, 84
Testosterone, 83, 84
Thermal energy, 59
Thermo labile, 77
Thermo stable, 79
Thiamin, 77
Thirsting, 91
Thrombosis, 146
Thuja, 133
Thymus, 85
Thyroid, 65, 85
Thyroxine, 65, 85
Tortoise, 37
Tomatoes, 66, 107, 108
Tongue, 154
Toxins, 25, 26, 27, 32, 40, 41, 44, 95, 107, 127
Trace elements, 41, 62, 67–72, 83
Trachea, 154
Treatment, 52
Tubercle baccilus, 66
Tuberculosis, 42, 155, 174
Turkish bath, 127
Turnips, 95, 98
Turtle, 37

U

Uncooked food, 118. 119
Ulceration, 42, 74, 78, 109, 159
Ultra sonic treatment, 173
Ultra violet treatment, 75, 172
Urea, 159
Urethra, 131
Uric acid, 92, 109, 159
Urinalysis, 158
Urine, 92, 158, 159

V

Vanadium, 68, 150
Vapour, 124
Vegans, 117
Vegetables, 54
Vegetarianism, 116–18
Vertebrae, 156
Vibration, 22, 24, 26, 41
Violet rays, 172
Virus, 42, 43, 81
Vital force, 20, 24, 25, 27, 29, 32, 33, 35, 36, 44, 48, 87
Vitamin "A", 60, 73, 74, 75
Vitamin "B$_1$", 77, 78
Vitamin "B$_2$", 77–8, 109
Vitamin "B$_6$", 78
Vitamin "B$_{12}$", 68
Vitamin "C", 80, 81, 82
Vitamin "D", 74–5
Vitamin "E", 75
Vitamin "H", 79
Vitamin "K", 75–6
Vitamin "P", 82
Vitamins, 41, 60, 63, 72–83, 109
Volt, 168
Voronoff, 83
Visual purple, 73

W

Waking, 177
Walnuts, 95
Wasting disease, 114
Watercress, 66, 98
Water, 2
Water soluble vitamins, 77–82
Water jet, 131
Water temperatures, 124
Water vapour, 124
Warts, 171
Watt, 169
Wet Pack, 91, 99, 131–3
Wheat, 66, 77
White wine, 92
Whiting, 116
Witch hazel, 136

Y

Yeast, 78, 80, 96
Yoghurt, 98, 112, 113
Youth, 35, 80, 83

Z

Zymotic, 144